Laughter, Tears and Braids

A father's journey through losing his wife to cancer

BRUCE HAM

D0873808

Laughter, Tears and Braids
Published through Publishing Unleashed

Interior Book Design and Layout by
www.integrativeink.com

ISBN: 978-0-9896359-0-5

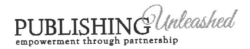

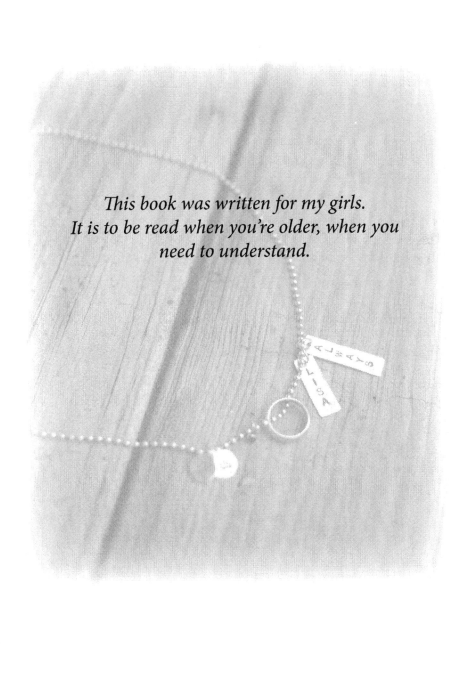

*This book was written for my girls.
It is to be read when you're older, when you
need to understand.*

Dear Bailey, Lucy and Annie T.,

I started writing the week after your mother got sick. Initially, it was in a journal given to me by a co-worker. At your uncle's urging, it turned into a blog, something I'd never heard of at the time. And now, after years of work, I have completed this book.

I'm not sure if anyone will read it; I'm not the best writer in the world. But that's not what this is about. I didn't write it to sell a million copies. I wrote it for you, I wrote it for Mom, and I wrote it for me.

You see, what your mother and I shared was beautiful. We loved each other very, very much. Throughout our 16-year marriage, we developed a connection and partnership I've never experienced before. In many ways, we were one.

She balanced me, and I brought out the best in her. Our strengths complemented each other. We filled each other's voids. I think that's why losing her was so difficult. Without her, I was lost. It was as if part of me had died too.

About halfway through putting this project together, I sat down and really thought about why I was writing. I wanted to make sure there was meaning in my work. I needed to know that this was more than just a reenactment of our life, a timeline of activities.

What I discovered was that the most important goal of this book is to help you better know your mother. I don't build her up to be perfect. She was not. She had incredible gifts and a few areas she could have improved upon – just like you and me.

You know me. You understand what I do well and what I don't. You love me for the good, and you give me grace for the bad. It's important that you know her too.

It is also important to me that you understand what your mother and I had together. We weren't the perfect couple; we were the perfect couple for us. I hope this book helps you have a picture of our marriage.

It was so very good. Maybe it will help you as you move forward in a serious relationship.

At times, I may have let you down during the year or two surrounding Mom's illness and death. It is important to me that you understand what was going in my mind at that time. I couldn't be all I should have been for you because I was simply broken – emotionally, physically and spiritually. I think I did okay, but at times I failed. You deserve to know why. You deserve to have a deeper understanding of the depth of my loss.

If anyone else reads this book, I hope they too will take something away.

For those who have experienced tragedy, I want them to see hope. I ached to the depths of my soul, and yet, even in my darkest days, there was happiness to be had – much of it I found in you.

I believe healing comes from within. It is all in how you play the cards you have been dealt. I'm no hero. I think that most people step up in the face of adversity, but maybe this book will help those who aren't yet able.

Finally, I hope to bring understanding to those who have not yet had to deal with loss. Perhaps a glimpse into our life will give them more understanding, more empathy for those walking through this long, hard journey. Truth be told, it's not just about death. There is sadness and strife all around, ours is but one example of how hard life can be.

I think this experience has made me appreciate what I have more than I ever did before. It has certainly changed my priorities. I wish I'd learned that sooner. Maybe others will read this and hug their kids a little tighter right now or take their wife out to dinner - tonight. That is my hope.

I don't think there is a way in words to express my love for the three of you. The pride and joy I feel for you exceeds even my own understanding. Without you, I'm not sure what would have happened to me. You provided me motivation to move forward when it would have been so easy to quit.

Take my words and forge on with life, regardless of the barriers that get put in your way. Reach out to those around you, showing acceptance, love and support, just as others have done for us; and, as you have done for me.

I love you.

Dad

Introduction

I was weak. I have been my entire life.

I'm not sure why. I don't think there is anything in particular that my parents did that caused me to be that way. Maybe it was just genetics.

I spent my entire life reliant on those around me for security and happiness. Perhaps most people do; I believe mine was just more extreme.

The first day of second grade, my mother walked me into Walker Spivey Elementary School in Fayetteville, NC. She didn't walk me in because she was a nervous mother. No, she walked me in because she was afraid; afraid I was going to refuse to stay.

She dropped me at Mrs. Hawk's class in mid-temper tantrum. I can imagine the thoughts running through my 7-year-old head: *If you think you're leaving my butt with these strangers, you're nuts!* As she walked down the hallway toward the front of the school where she'd parked, I bolted out the back door of my classroom. I'm not sure if my teacher saw me. I don't recall her on my trail.

When my mother arrived at our blue Plymouth station wagon, with the brown-paneled sides, parked in the front circle of the school, she was surprised to find me in the passenger seat, proud of my own cunning.

I'm not sure why she was so surprised. The year prior I had attended a school two blocks from our house. As my older brother, Chad, and our caravan of friends walked me to school, I embraced the fire hydrant refusing to let go. It took my mother, brother and two of Chad's friends to pry me free. Fortunately for my mom, Mrs. Brayboy was my teacher. She cracked a kid's fingers on the first day of school for chatting too much. I could only imagine what she'd do to me if I ran out of her classroom door.

This pattern of insecurity continued throughout my life. Although I became less likely to physically hold onto neighborhood fixtures, my desire to be in the comfort of my own home didn't cease until my second try at college. My first ended after three weeks and with my car crammed full of my belongings. I think my father was as surprised to see me that Sunday afternoon in 1983, as my mother was in the station wagon in 1972. Perhaps he thought maybe this time I'd give him some space, some time alone with my mom. Not so. I was 17, and it would be another year before I was ready to venture out on my own.

I grew as I aged, eventually marrying and becoming a father. My happiness, however, was never found from within. The foundation of my outer confidence was not based on my own success. It centered on the strength of those around me. I would be taken care of first by my parents and then by my wife. They built me up; they held me together.

My insecurities weren't evident to the world. I didn't always realize I had them. I had a great job and was a pretty good father. I was involved in my community and a leader at church. But my wife was my strength. I had never felt comfortable as just me. I felt comfortable as us.

She was my rock, the base of my statue. What would I do when it crumbled apart?

Chapter 1

August 2009

Capon Springs, West Virginia, is nestled in a valley directly over the Virginia line about an hour and forty-five minutes from Washington, DC. Capon is like the old movie *Brigadoon*. You return annually and the place is exactly the same as when you left. The same people return year after year, a bit older, perhaps a bit wider or balder, but return they do. My mother-in-law grew up in Fairmont, West Virginia, and first visited Capon in 1949. Over sixty years later, the family's fondness for the place has remained the same.

If you marry into Capon, it takes years to get your footing. Years. But for those born into a Capon family, the love for the place is instantaneous. My wife, Lisa, vacationed at Capon the third week in August all thirty-nine years of her life. So I did too.

I'm not sure what makes Capon so special. The accommodations are sparse. Our room, and it is our room for life if we choose, has one double bed and one twin. The furniture is identical to the bedroom set from my childhood room in Fayetteville, North Carolina. There's a small wooden nightstand with one drawer and a small 40-watt bulbed lamp nailed to the wall above the bed, its light tan shade always askew. A sink protrudes from the wall, a mirror hangs over it no bigger than my head. A bottle opener that was screwed on the door in the 1960s remains neatly in place, although I can't remember a time we've used it over the years. There's no air conditioning, no Wi-Fi, no TV. A shared bathroom sits at the end of the hall, 93 steps from my room. I've counted them many times over the years when I relieved myself in the middle of the night.

Every day at 8 am sharp, the two hundred guests gather at the flagpole outside of the main house. Lisa always stood proudly in the middle. Yes, she was in the middle — of everything. I always straggle in late, a step behind, at least one kid in tow.

Once the crowd is assembled, the music begins, and the chosen child for the day raises the flag. The tape of a woman, with a vibrato that could challenge the best soprano in any Southern Baptist Church choir, belts out "The land of the free" and holds it long enough to shatter crystal glasses in Wardensville, ten miles away.

My father-in-law David, a stout attorney with a fairly stubborn edge, works hard to woo the attention of our three daughters, but to no avail. At Capon they are free — free to roam with their annual playmates. There is no time for those they see back home.

We then move into the dining room for a family-style home-cooked breakfast with eggs any way you want them.

One year, I decided I would order a different kind of egg each day that week: boiled, scrambled, sunny side up, over easy, over light, over hard, poached. It didn't rattle our waitress, Charlotte. She's been serving our family for a decade or more. Charlotte knows Lisa's brother wants extra whip cream on Friday night with his apple crisp. She brings a huge bowl to the table without him even requesting it.

During the day we play golf and tennis. A spring-fed pool with horseflies that draw blood sits at a chilly 68 degrees. Heat it? Absurd! It's never been heated. They call it refreshing. I call it sterilizing. It took me six years and two kids to dip below my thighs. For a guy, the step from thigh to belly button is significant.

On Saturday night, the culmination of the week's activities occurs after dinner, the mixed doubles shuffle board tournament finals. Matches are played all week until the final two pairs meet. In our family, Lisa and her younger, and only, brother Hayes were always partners. Her father and her younger sister, Sallie, another annual pair. My mother-in-law and Sallie's husband Matt join in about every other year. "Our family is just not committed" my competitive father-in-law tells us. His theory is to put off playing your matches as long as you possibly can. That way you can continue to tout that you're "still in" for a longer period of time. Intimidation tactic? Perhaps. Although he's shared his theory with most of the old school Caponeers so I'm not sure it's still effective.

One year Sallie and David won the finals. Lisa and Hayes made it into the final round in the early 2000s, but did not come home with the prized apple butter. Lisa said she would rather have the second place prize anyway, homemade chocolate chip cookies. It is difficult to beat the Fitzpatrick family, who take the game very seriously. One year when the Fitzpatrick patriarch got on his granddaughter about her shuffleboard tourney performance, Lisa jumped to her rescue. Perhaps it was none of her business, but a gutsy call nonetheless. Not at all unexpected from my wife. All the other guests talked about that "exchange" for the remainder of the night. It was big news: a 30-year-old-woman confronting a 70-year-old man. And the Czar of Capon shuffleboard at that!

Lisa wasn't scared of Frank Fitzpatrick. In fact, Lisa wasn't really scared of anything. She wasn't demanding; if she paid too much for something that should have been on sale, she wouldn't raise a stink. She wasn't one to complain to a manager about a lousy waitress. Her attitude was, she's lousy but she probably has a hard life. It's no big deal. But if she believed in something, you'd better get out of her way.

She believed in our annual family vacations to Capon Springs. I might have suggested we take the two grand we spend at Capon each year and use it for a different adventure. Blasphemy! I quickly learned that marrying Lisa meant a lifelong commitment to spending each August in the place that never changes.

I can tell you what I will eat on Thursdays the third week in August for the rest of my life. For breakfast, scrambled eggs (if I choose), scrapple, buckwheat pancakes and cocoa wheat. Twice each week, Thursday included, Capon staff serve dinner on the Hill, a covered pavilion on the first hole fairway. There is grilled steak and ham, burgers and dogs, corn on the cob, butter beans, rolls and sweet tea. To top this spread off, blueberry pie a la mode! I anticipate dinner on the Hill the first part of the week and work to stretch my stomach for the feast that's ahead. I also plan to stand or lay down for the rest of Thursday night. It's difficult to sit after a four-meat dinner.

Because the guests depend on Capon for consistency, change does not come easily. If I wanted a new brand of soap, I'd just go to the store and buy a different bar. When Capon went from bars to soft soap in a dispenser in each shower, there was hell to pay! Lisa and her girl-friends, most of whom have been coming to Capon for multiple years, had plenty to say about that.

Lisa headed up the gossip mill the third week in August. She kept a list of the guests in our car and would review their names and any sordid history that accompanied them on the five-hour drive from Raleigh. Once there, she would exercise her God-given ability to talk, she was the master, with various allies at the many venues throughout the resort.

I'd catch her at the pool with our friend, Jeannette, discussing who had come in after curfew the night before. She and her lifelong buddy, Emily, would walk a batch of kids to the hog farm, Hog Heaven, a few miles down the road. It wasn't for the exercise or for the chance to see a live pig; instead, a chance to talk.

"We're going to let the kids see the hogs," she'd say before leaving.

"You're going to run your mouths," I'd retort.

She'd roll her eyes and begin her conversation. There were more pressing matters to discuss.

I'll have to admit I liked sleeping with the leading member of the Capon CIA. She had information that any spy would kill for. And because of our close relationship and her loose lips, I knew it all.

Because of the amount of food intake at Capon, I spend quite a bit of time in my third floor bathroom. Although it is shared with ten other guys, I don't mind. Over the years I've figured out their bathroom habits and know exactly when the stalls are clear.

One year at Capon, Annie T., our third child who was a precocious four-year-old at the time, devised a new system for categorizing our bathroom habits. We'd always used number 1 for pee and number 2 for poop. I was in the main house living room talking with a group of friends when Annie T. ran up and said, "I have to go number 5." Naturally I became curious.

"Number 5?"

"Yes, peepee *and* poopies," she emphasized the *and*.

"Are there more?"

"Number 1 is pee pee. Number 2 is EMergency pee pee (emphasis on the EM). Number 3 is poopie. Number 4 is EMergency poopie. Number 5 is pee pee AND poopie. And Number 6 is diarrhea."

Ed Offtendinger, a svelte 50-year-old balding man who was clearly an athlete in his day, overheard our conversation. He grimly suggested that there was also room for a zero on this scale. From the look on his face, the food was catching up with him. It was Thursday, right after dinner on the hill.

Lisa was a consistent zero. So by the middle of our Capon week in 2009, spending a significant amount of time in the bathroom for her was unusual. Even the third week in August didn't typically call for her normal routine to change.

Lisa wasn't a particularly healthy person, but she wasn't unhealthy. She didn't exercise, and she had Type II Diabetes, but she ate well and saw her doctor on a regular basis. And she certainly wasn't one to complain.

She told me that when she was a kid it took an Act of Congress to miss school. Her memory was that she and her siblings had to have fever over 104 and be vomiting with significant diarrhea for a doctor's visit. I, on the other hand, could cough and say, "I don't feel good" and my mom would call an ambulance. The principal at Glendale Acres Elementary School kept a bottle of Emotrol in his office to relax my always upset stomach.

If you were the first one drilled in the chest during German dodge ball by Scotty Cannon on the playground daily, you'd have an upset stomach too. Scotty had hair on his chest in the third grade and scared the crap out of me.

Lisa had some stomach problems prior to this visit to Capon. Later that fall she shared with me that at her annual physical in September of 2008, the doctor asked if she had any issues she wanted to discuss. Lisa thought a minute and responded, "My husband says that I always say my stomach is upset. I hadn't really noticed it myself but as I think about it, I have had some discomfort." The doctor asked a few more questions and discovered that her stomach wasn't affecting Lisa at the moment, so they decided to monitor things and touch base if she developed a pattern or other significant symptoms.

Although I vaguely remember telling my wife she complained often about her stomach, my first significant recollection of specific gastric issues for Lisa was in early 2009, about four months after that doctor's appointment. We attributed her discomfort to the fact that she had begun to drink coffee after refraining for the summer and fall. She stopped again, and immediately felt better.

That winter passed without another flare up. We had four week-long vacations planned for the spring and summer of that year including Capon. There was no time to deal with intestinal issues. Life was too short for the inconvenience and there were no signs of serious illness. The symptoms were sporadic; there was little that could be done at that time, we thought.

No one in our family spent a lot of time at the doctor's office but we did occasionally use Lisa's sister for an over the phone diagnosis. Sallie graduated from John's Hopkins with a PhD in epidemiology and from Harvard with an MD. You'd think she'd be of significant help when a family member gets sick. She is not. She loathes diagnosing family illnesses, perhaps because the diseases she sees in the hospital are far more dangerous and interesting. Once my brother-in-law, at age 22, had his tonsils removed. When Hayes began coughing up blood two days later and called Sallie, she said, "Well, I don't know what it is — just keep an eye on it and if it gets worse, call the doctor."

"I thought I just did," he whispered through his raw throat.

He could have just called me for that diagnosis, and I'm a director at the local YMCA.

Sallie's a smart lady who infects monkeys for a living. She publishes all kinds of findings on her research on AIDS in children in Africa. In many ways she is a genius. In other ways, she is not.

At one point in her younger days, Sallie's language consisted primarily of the words "whatever" and "like." One Christmas our family was reading scripture at the Christmas Eve service. We were practicing, but Sallie wasn't home from school yet. So we decided to read the Christmas story as if we were Sallie.

> *Like there was this girl named Mary, and she rode a donkey— seriously?—to Bethlehem to birth the Messiah. And she was a virgin, as if. That's not exactly possible. I'm a scientist and you really can't have a baby without sperm. But anyway, she had to stay in a stable with animals—gross! When the baby came out they wrapped him in swaddling clothes and cinched it in the middle with a nice belt from the Gap.*

She applied for Medical School at several places. One of them was Harvard, another was Yale. She told us that after a long day of interviewing at Yale all of the applicants joined the faculty for dinner at a trendy restaurant. There she had an E.F. Hutton moment. Everyone was talking and someone asked her if she liked the town. She said, "Yeah, I love it! It even has a Gap!" And as the words were rolling out of her mouth, everyone at the table stopped talking and looked directly at her, disapprovingly. You can tell by their style that the academic crowd isn't spending a lot of time at the Gap, or any other non-thrift store. She did not get in. But I guess if you are accepted at Harvard, rejection from Yale is not that big of a letdown.

Because of Sallie's lack of interest in diagnosing family illnesses, I was surprised that when Lisa's stomach began giving her trouble at Capon, Sallie readily accompanied her to the bathroom. What they discovered was that Lisa's stool was very dark. Sallie was concerned enough that Lisa immediately set an appointment for a colonoscopy in Raleigh for the following Friday.

After setting the appointment, her intestines didn't cross my mind again until the day of her procedure. I had golf to play, fried chicken to eat and a shuffle board tournament to watch. Everyone has stomach problems now and then.

Chapter 2

Spring 1990

I first fell in love with Lisa on a canoe at the YMCA's Camp Seafarer. Camp Seafarer is a girls' overnight sailing camp located in Arapahoe on the North Carolina coast. We both worked at the Y in Raleigh with a group of middle school kids who met every Wednesday afternoon and Saturday morning. I began working as a Y Youth Counselor when I was still in college. I worked every Saturday morning from 8 am –noon and looking back on it am amazed that I held down a job that required an early weekend morning commitment.

I became the Youth Director at the Y in my early twenties. It was 1989. Lisa was still a college student at The University of North Carolina - Chapel Hill. She would make the 30-minute drive from school to Raleigh on some Saturdays to help me supervise the kids. I'm proud to say that I was her boss. Had I known I would end up marrying her, I would have spent more time savoring that short-lived role.

On one Saturday morning around 1990, I distinctly remember leaving a child at McDonalds. At that time, there was no Vice President of Risk Management at the Y. There were no guidelines to follow. If we decided to take the kids to McDonalds in our cars, we took them. This time there were 17 teens. Lisa was 20-years-old and drove seven of the kids in her mother's blue station wagon that had a third row back seat that faced the rear of the vehicle. I drove the rest in the Y van. This van had a stench that would curl your hair. There were always single socks in the van. Old, nasty, sweaty athletic socks left under the seat; odd that there was always a single, but never a pair. I can still remember the smell, like cooked cabbage and my dad after a good day of yard work combined.

We drove to the McDonald's on Peace Street near downtown and everyone unloaded. It is interesting how much fast food and pizza we ate in the youth department at the Y in those days. The YMCA was an organization that was known worldwide for its fitness programs and yet, one year in the 1990s we ate $21,000 worth of pizza at one Y branch.

That morning the kids ordered their food, followed by a second trip to the cashier for a McFluffy or whatever the sundae with chocolate syrup in the plastic cup with the hole in the lid was called. We all, well all but one, piled back in the two vehicles and drove back to the Y on Hillsborough Street as their parents arrived in the carpool line to pick up their kids.

Car number 8 was a problem. We knew the parent well. José was of Hispanic descent, one of only two kids in the program who wasn't lily, country club, white. We called for José, no response. We checked the bathroom, no José; the auditorium, no José. I made a quick sweep through the gym, checked the youth locker rooms and the bottom of the pool; looking back on it, we should have checked there first. I was headed to the men's locker room for one last ditch effort at finding the kid when Lisa called me on the walkie-talkie: "José called. We left him at McDonald's. His dad has gone to get him. He's not happy."

"Who's not happy?" I said.

"The father," she replied.

"Crap!"

We could handle an unhappy kid. And I was all about sweet-talking the moms. But a mad father was bound to land me in my boss's office on Monday morning.

In my defense, this group of teens was an odd assortment of misfits. None were very cool; all were very funny. There was Tim, the rotund African American kid who lived down the street from the Y. "Rerun" comes to mind. Bill was a thin boy working to figure out his sexuality.

He wore skirts to the Y and often painted his fingernails pink. David Pizzotti was a kid who one day on a teen trip to the grocery store picked up a half gallon of red wine and put it in the cart. "I got your jug of wine, Bruuuuce."

"Put the wine back now, Pizzotti, now!"

Eli was a pudgy kid with glasses who resembled Queen Elizabeth. We had two girls in the program, and they were actually pretty normal. Lisa was charged with looking after them. I was charged with Pizzotti and the motley gang of 15.

Monday came and went with no phone call from José's dad — or at least if he called, my boss did not relay the message to me. He was back the next week too. I think his father was just thankful to get José out of the house for four hours on a Saturday morning, and I didn't blame him.

Once a year, as a fundraiser, we would take the kids down to Camp Seafarer to work in the kitchen for the weekend camp guests. After leaving a kid at McDonald's earlier in the year, I should have been more tentative about asking Lisa to chaperone this trip with me. But I needed backup and there weren't a lot of takers. Besides, I liked the fact that Lisa was a strong youth counselor, as we called them, and a talker. She didn't take any junk from the boys. Anything they dished out, she threw right back at them. And the same was true for me. I asked her if she'd be responsible for "wet garbage" — basically the leftovers off of everyone's plate dropped into a large rolling trash can. Her response? "I'll take care of the silverware." Any other youth counselor working for me, male or female, would have done exactly what I asked them to do. Not Lisa. She knew she was getting paid whether she slopped wet garbage or set the tables for the next meal, and she wasn't about to touch food that had potentially been in someone else's mouth. Although daring and strong, I would soon find out that she was also a refined woman who sported manicured nails, liked high heels and expensive clothes, and, she really didn't toot. I couldn't see all of this then, but what I did see, I liked.

After sweating over half-eaten bacon, eggs, and pancakes and setting tables for 600 guests, the kids headed out to the camp activities for several hours of free time. I, clearly with some attraction to Lisa, asked her if she wanted to go relax in Taylor Lodge, one of the only air-conditioned spots at camp. She agreed. I took off my shirt and escorted her to the canoe dock. "Can't we walk?" she asked.

"This way is shorter." I gestured to the canoe. *And more romantic,* I thought to myself. She rolled her eyes and sat down. I don't know what it was about her, but at that moment, she stole my heart.

Chapter 3

September 4, 2009

Lisa and I had a great deal in common which may have initially brought us together. We both had strong political convictions and a similar outlook on God and religion. We were both headstrong, outgoing and gregarious. But there were some differences that we'd have to contend with.

I was a yard man. I could spend all weekend cutting, blowing, mowing and edging. Lisa seldom went outside, unless it was to get into her car to drive to the mall. I loved to exercise. Lisa, not so much; in fact, not at all. My wife could talk to a tree for hours. She knew everyone in town, their children's names, their birthdays and who their second cousin was. I called our neighbor Stavrulla for years, simply because I couldn't remember her name. When this neighbor first moved in, Lisa asked me her name because I was the first to meet her.

"I can't remember. It was something like Stavrulla."

"Are you serious? Stavrulla?"

"Don't quote me on it, but it's something like that."

A few weeks later, Lisa came storming into the house. "Guess who I saw today?"

"I have no idea."

"I saw Stavrulla. But guess what?"

"What?"

"Her name is Katrina."

"Oh, that's a nice name."

"How in the world did you get Stavrulla from Katrina?"

"I don't know. She just looks like a Stavrulla to me."

"That's what a Stavrulla looks like? What if I had called her that?"

"You'd have been embarrassed."

"And you would have been dead," she quipped.

My wife had a way of looking at me. It was a mix of disgust, wonder and delight all rolled up in one.

"I am married to a moron."

Lisa was laidback; nothing really bothered her except calling the neighbor by the wrong name. That included her "roll with the punches" outlook on her medical issues. When we discovered she developed gestational diabetes with our first child, she was required to drink this thick, sugary liquid and have her blood checked every 15 minutes for three hours. I waited with her in the lobby of the doctor's office and almost passed out just watching from 10 yards away. I DO NOT LIKE NEEDLES digging into my veins! I don't give blood. If blood ever comes out of me, I have had an accident or it is being forcibly taken.

After sitting through Lisa's three-hour diabetes ordeal, I promised never to have sex with her again. I didn't want to risk getting her pregnant and requiring more needles. But drawing blood and medical issues didn't rattle Lisa. The day before the appointment that she and Sallie set while on vacation at Capon required her to drink what seemed like 32 gallons of thick wash-your-innards out juice for a colonoscopy. As usual, she was a good sport.

I've never seen anyone go to the bathroom as much as she did the night before she went to have her colon photographed. She ran, I mean ran, to the pot several times in a panic. It was actually quite entertaining. By the end of the night, her poop was clearer than rum.

Our family's lack of fear about the possibility of Lisa having something seriously wrong with her was evident by the email exchanges between Lisa, her sister, brother and me in the days before her colonoscopy.

Sallie: *I call Lisa for the family Christmas gift exchange this year! I have lots of potty/poop-related items in mind. Sam [Sallie's infant son] will put together a collection of his favorite poopy diapers for her too. (Bruce told me to say it!)*

Me: I DID NOT. Her poop is off limits for me. I have pledged not to make any jokes about her colon…and except for putting together a care package for her the other night (had each kid go find something potty-related to put by her bed – magazine, plunger, t. paper, crossword puzzle), I have done well.

Hayes: What's up with Lisa's colon? And if she gets it -oscopied is there anything we can get bronzed? Or how about poo-wtered? [this was in reference to their mother giving her children their baby shoes dipped in pewter the previous Christmas].

Sallie: Poo-tered! I laughed so hard I nearly peed in my pants. For once it is not me as the "butt" of the joke!

Me: She's been having a lot of stomach issues. They are ruling things out. Probably much doo doo about nothing.

Lisa: I'm not coming to Christmas.

The next morning I had to drive to Camp Seafarer on business. We had arranged for Lisa's mother to take her for the procedure.

Although I'd seen Lisa "prepping" for hours the night before, her colon did not cross my mind the entire day. I spent hours in meetings, had a chicken salad sandwich at the country club in Arapahoe for lunch and enjoyed a day of work in the setting where I had originally fallen in love with my wife.

On the way back from camp, I remembered that she had the appointment late that afternoon. I called less out of concern and more out of obligation. It seemed no more important to me than if she had been scheduled for a root canal.

I was in Goldsboro, North Carolina, about an hour from the house when her mother picked up Lisa's cell phone. This was a conversation that was unfortunately repeated several times over the next few months of my life. One that I grew to abhor.

"So how's the patient?" I asked, fully expecting a rote, "*She's fine.*"

Ann hesitated, "She's OK."

"How was the colonoscopy?"

"Well," pause, "we're still here."

"Is something wrong?"

"Lisa, Bruce wants to know if something is wrong. Do you want to talk to him? Let me get Lisa." Although I'd never had the phone passed in the same manner before, I sensed we had a problem.

Lisa picked up with a groggy voice, "Honey, I just woke up. The nurses are in the room. Just come home; we'll talk then."

"OK, baby. You alright?"

"Just come home."

The phone went silent.

My mind went nuts: *Oh my God! My wife has cancer. She's going to die. I'll be alone. It's over. I just told my buddy from work that we had the best summer of our life. I have cursed us.*

I called my mom.

"Mom, Lisa just had her colonoscopy, and they have found something. I think it's cancer."

"How do you know?"

"I don't. But the nurses were all in the room, and she said she couldn't talk right now. It's got to be bad."

"Honey, you're jumping to conclusions. There are all sorts of things they can find in a colonoscopy. It is probably something else."

"What else can they find?"

"Well, let me think. Wayne, Bruce wants to know what else they can find in a colonoscopy other than cancer. What can you tell him?" I heard my dad stammering.

"You got nothing, Mom. It's definitely cancer."

"No honey, it could be Irritable Bowel Syndrome, Crohn's Disease; there are multiple things it could be."

If your hair were on fire, my mother could find a way to tell you it looked nice and that everything would be OK. As a nerdy high school student who stunk at athletics, I struggled with self-esteem. But my mother made me feel like I was Brad Pitt. She constantly talked about how handsome I was, how smart I was and how creative and capable I was.

The rest of the drive was tough.

When I arrived home, I found Lisa sitting in a chair by the back door. Her legs were folded Indian style under her lap. She was wearing a pair of black stretchy pants with a matching black and white jacket. Her eyes were swollen. She had been crying.

Her mother was standing and ready to go. She needed some time to process and obsess without Lisa in the room. Lisa said, through tears, "It's cancer."

I liken that short sentence to being punched in the stomach by Mike Tyson…in his prime. It hurt from my testicles to my chest. My body and my heart sank. I was floored.

I called my parents to tell them what they found: a tumor so large that they couldn't get the adult scope in her colon; they had to use the pediatric scope.

I went to the porch and called my best friend Brad who I work with. I struggled to get the words out. "How could this be? She's 39 years old. We have three daughters. This can't be." Maybe it's not that serious, I tried to convince myself. But a pediatric scope? It's big. It's bad. It's going to get her.

Lisa Update, 9-4-09
To: Co-workers
From: Bruce

Dear Friends,

Been a tough day. We just found out that Lisa has colon cancer. We don't have many specifics right now—all is new with few answers. We go to see the surgeon on Tuesday morning. I may or may not be in that day. We think she will have significant surgery and pretty fast. That is about all we know at this point.

Please keep us in your thoughts and prayers. Raw to talk about right now.

Bruce

My general life's philosophy is to assume the worst and be surprised. That instinct took over. I assumed she'd be gone by Christmas, and I wasn't far off.

Chapter 4

1990 – 1991

I had dated a number of women in my life; some for short periods of time, some for years. I'd never been the most attractive guy on the block, a stick for a body with the exception of slight love handles. I was a funny, steady soul with sufficient insecurities, not much of a risk taker. Cool would not be a word that was used to describe me.

I'm not really sure what a girl ever saw in me. But there never seemed to be a shortage. I'll have to admit, I really didn't treat them very well. These women weren't the most beautiful women in the world, but they certainly weren't ugly. I think they stuck with me because they just wanted to settle down, and I appeared to be the good settling kind.

At times it was as if they didn't have minds of their own. They let me make all of the decisions in our relationships. I always called the shots.

I seldom dated one at a time. My mantra was: one on the front burner, one on the back burner and one walking by the stove. I wasn't dishonest with the women I dated. They knew I was spending time with others, and they seemingly didn't care enough to break things off. That was not, however, the woman I wanted to marry. I wanted someone independent. Someone who would say, "Hell, no you're not dating anyone else! You can kiss my behind, Bruce Ham." And that's just what I found in Lisa.

When I returned home from Camp Seafarer after chaperoning our motley crew of teens with Lisa, I was absolutely smitten. I was so attracted to her; I couldn't get her out of my head. She knew I was interested but proceeded to spend the summer juggling two other guys, not giving me the time of day.

In the summer of 1990, Lisa ran the pool for the summer day camp at the downtown YMCA in Raleigh. I was still the Youth Director there and once again, her supervisor. This was about two months after we'd chaperoned together at Camp Seafarer.

Lisa was nice enough at work, but when 6 pm hit, she was out the door. She had a long-time crush on a frat boy she dated at the UNC. He was in Raleigh for the summer, and she worked that relationship hard.

I called him by his last name, Tisdale, and pronounced it with the same disdain that Seinfeld used when referring Newman. I still hate that guy. In addition to Tisdale, I found out she was spending time with a fellow camp counselor named Charlie. Although I liked him a lot, I could not for the life of me figure out how in the heck he was more attractive to Lisa than I. He was about as interesting as a sheep and equaled me in the looks department. I believe she had a plan; a plan to harness me — and Charlie was retained simply to draw me into her trap. The more she ignored me, the more I wanted to be with her. I dated other women that summer, but my mind was on her the entire time.

She returned to school that fall. I thought about her often but struggled to figure out a strategy for running into her. What excuse could I have to be in Chapel Hill? I was a graduate of NC State, an arch rival of UNC. There was nothing there I needed —nothing except Lisa.

When one thinks of the town of Chapel Hill, one thinks of the University of North Carolina. It is a nationally-recognized school, a college town, and that's about all. So, what could I do? Go back to school? Ridiculous.

After a fall of not being able to get Lisa off my mind, I enrolled in continuing education at UNC under the guise that I might return to graduate school to fulfill a lifelong dream of obtaining a master's degree. I didn't even know what I might be getting that degree in - perhaps communication? I liked to communicate. A master's degree could help. I registered for an early morning class on Tuesdays and Thursdays for the spring semester of 1991. I called Lisa and asked her if she'd like to meet me on Thursday mornings before class to grab breakfast and discuss the upcoming summer camp program. She had agreed to return to the Y for one more year; how could she tell her boss no?

Each Thursday, we met at her dorm and drove to Ye Ole Waffle Shoppe on Franklin Street where we had some great conversations. An hour of catching up. An hour of getting to know each other better. Not a lot of talk about summer camp, although I probably turned the receipt in to work just to clear my guilty conscience.

I was convinced she was beginning to be attracted to me until April 19, 1991. I drove into Chapel Hill at the usual time, 7:15 am. I parked in the usual place right outside of Cobb Dorm. And there I waited. And waited. And waited. I couldn't get into the dorm, it was all female and the doors were locked. We did not have cell phones back then, so I couldn't call. I had no way to get in touch with her. I didn't know what to do. I had never been stood up before in my entire life. I had been the stander upper —not the standee. I was pissed.

At around 7:45, I fumed all the way to Ye Ole Waffle Shoppe. I fumed over my four cups of coffee. I couldn't concentrate in class. I said to myself, *I am not a toy! I will NOT be treated like this. I am through with that woman. I am done!* I returned to the Y in Raleigh and announced to the two women I worked with, one of them a very close friend of Lisa's, "I am through with Lisa Permar! I am NOT a toy."

Lisa and I talked later that day, and I found out that she had celebrated her 21st birthday on April 18, and being the party girl that she was, it was a memorable night. She drank too much, got into bed late and actually sprained her ankle pretty badly. I hated that for her, but I had decided I was through. I had chased her for a year; she had dominated my thoughts for 12 months, and I was done. I was not going to be taken advantage of, waiting around for her, like the many women I had dated over the years. I would simply return to my stove-top dating philosophy, and Lisa Permar would be put on the back burner.

Chapter 5

Lisa Update: 9-5-09
To: Friends and Family
From: Lisa

Dear Friends,

I am writing to let you know of a diagnosis that I received Friday which is easier to share over email than in person. If you have been lucky enough to have been spared my recent issues, then this will be really out of the blue—

I was diagnosed on Friday with colon cancer. I will meet with a surgeon on Tuesday to schedule the removal of a tumor. I will not know any other details of the cancer (stage, treatment, etc) until the surgery is performed.

My medical team today included 3 women, all current or former St. Timothy's [the school where Lisa worked] moms. It was nice to have familiar faces around me. They were all shocked with their findings, as my age and family history would not have led them to predict this outcome.

I suspect the surgery will be scheduled quickly and I was told I should expect at least a week of recovery. We have told the kids and used the word cancer, focusing on the removal of the tumor and not the potential steps after that. Annie T. already wants to know if I need to have my head shaved.

I do not mind my diagnosis being shared—it's easier for you to share it with others than for me to do it. But, as most of you know, I often wear my emotions on my sleeve and I don't want to be a blubbering idiot for the next few weeks. So keep the humor and the distractions coming. Isn't there a quote from Steel Magnolias about laughter through tears being the best emotion? I imagine you'll see a lot of that from me—so keep the tissues handy when in my presence!

Thanks for your prayers and patience as we navigate whatever lies ahead.

Lisa

The first doctor we met with was at Rex Hospital, five minutes from our house. He told us that Lisa had colon cancer and that he would do surgery immediately. He said he would remove the tumor and sew her colon back together. Then, she would receive radiation and chemo. He was ready to move the following week.

Lisa and I weren't really ones to rock the boat. The doctor who performed the colonoscopy recommended this surgeon and Rex was a very good hospital with a strong reputation. We were ready to move. However, Sallie had a different plan.

As a Harvard graduate and an infectious disease specialist at Boston Children's Hospital, Sallie felt strongly that we needed to consider care from Duke or Chapel Hill, both associated with a medical school, both less than 30 minutes from our house and renowned for cancer care.

As Sallie began talking with her colleagues, it seemed that for colon cancer all roads led to Duke. Thanks to Sallie, we had an appointment the day after we met with the doctor at Rex.

When we entered the Duke waiting room, it was sort of like going to a doctor's version of Walmart. Unlike Rex where there was a nice waiting room with plenty of seating, Duke packed them in like sardines. I could not believe we were sitting on the floor in a waiting room that was full of people with cancer. A little old lady came by with a cup of Coke and some packaged cookies. She looked like David Letterman's mother. We declined her kind offer.

I was a snob. I didn't like to wait. I didn't like crowds. I didn't like people breathing all in my space. I didn't like Coke poured in a cup out of a liter bottle that is shared by a bunch of people I didn't know with germs significant enough to warrant a hospital visit. I was ready to go back to Rex — because it was more comfortable *for me*.

Lisa and I got tickled looking at the people. All different ages, shapes and sizes. We were on the younger end of the spectrum. There were people all over the place like mosquitoes on a baby.

When we finally got called back and met with the surgeon, Dr. Tyler, he said he wanted to examine Lisa. He told us that he had a feeling this tumor was lower in the colon, bordering on rectal cancer. Lisa asked how he knew. He said, "I just know."

His tone was both grave and reassuring. I could tell from his demeanor that he wasn't playing games — this was serious. And yet, his confidence led me to believe he knew exactly what he was doing.

When Lisa returned from the examining room, she described her experience.

"He took at hard straw and stuck it up my ass. Then, he invited everyone in the doctor's office to look up my crack. Seriously, there were eight students in line to look into the scope. And every one of them eyeballed the tumor in my rear end."

As the "class" entered the room, apparently Lisa said, "Looks like the gang's all here! Come on in and take a look." I don't think they saw the humor. She saw humor in a lot of things.

When Dr. Tyler returned to our room, he explained that Lisa had a very large tumor near the bottom of the colon. He called it colorectal cancer, but we didn't like that word so we just called it colon cancer.

He drew a picture with his Bic pen on the paper that covered the small bed in the room. He explained that with colorectal cancer you typically began with a series of radiation treatments, about 12 weeks, along with a low dose of chemo. Surgery would follow and then strong chemotherapy for six months. He told us Lisa would have a temporary ileostomy bag after surgery. Months after chemo, if there were no further signs of cancer, they would reconstruct her intestines, and the bag would be removed.

As he spoke, I wept. Lisa held it together, because that's what Lisa did. She had the ability to attack this head on without wallowing in fear. This woman I had married had grit. As I dissolved from the news, she asked about next steps.

A CAT scan was set for the next day.

We held hands the entire ride home. We both cried, but didn't talk much. What was there to say?

Lisa Update, 9-9-09
To: Friends and Family
From: Lisa

Spent an exhausting afternoon at Duke, and they have turned me upside down. Totally different approach to the treatment than Rex. We are looking at something more serious than Stage 1 cancer. Their approach is to start chemo and radiation and then to do surgery. I will be at Duke all day tomorrow. First at the lab, then in radiology and then meeting with radiation and oncology together.

It is amazing how much more these people seemed to know than everything else we have heard and read. This is a whole new ball game and we are adjusting our thinking.

We don't need anything at this time but we'll let you know when we do.

Lisa

Journal Entry 9-10-09

> CT scan. <u>*Ovary enlarged.*</u>
> *Lung clear—praise God*
> *Liver clear—praise God*
> *Bones clear—praise God*
> *Bad, sad day*

On September 11, seven days after we found out Lisa had cancer, we found ourselves in the office of Dr. Lee, an OBGYN oncologist. Lisa had a good attitude and bounced into the lobby and began a welcoming conversation with the receptionist. She explained her situation and signed in for the appointment. Her optimism helped to minimize my anxiety.

Dr. Lee was a short Asian lady, I think. I never really saw her face. She wore a mask the entire visit. She could have been an impersonator, no one would have known.

She was very businesslike. I'm sure she was as excited about seeing us as we were about seeing her. People don't really smile at you when you first find out you have cancer. Signs of humor and levity seemed to imply an attitude of flippancy. It wasn't that Lisa didn't take this seriously; it was that she refused to allow adversity to squelch her love for life.

The masked doctor informed us that she wanted to do an exam to check for endometrial cancer and asked me to leave the room. I should have questioned her.

Instead I went to the lobby as instructed and lost my already shaky composure.

Now we may have THREE cancers? The colon is definite, her ovary is enlarged, and now we're checking for endometrial? Holy shit! I can't keep up with them all. Maybe it would be easier to make a list of the cancers that she does NOT have.

I held my head in my hands. For the first time, I really felt that her days here on earth were limited. I was in that lobby for what seemed like hours. I was beside myself. I couldn't focus. I couldn't retain a concrete thought.

The nurse called me back into the room. I immediately asked Dr. Lee, "What makes you suspect she has endometrial cancer?"

"Oh, I don't suspect that. It is doubtful. And if she does have it, it is very slow growing and is the least of your worries. It's just a simple test, so I wanted to do it while she was here."

"So you don't think she has endometrial cancer?"

"I don't think so. I'm just ruling it out."

We may only have two cancers!!! WHOA. WHOA.

We called Lisa's dad and met him at the PR, a local bar, to celebrate with a pitcher of beer. I never dreamed I'd be happy that we were only dealing with two cancers. It was an indicator of how poorly things were going.

Chapter 6

Fall, 1991

After the 21st birthday incident, Lisa and I played cat and mouse for the next two years. One weekend in 1991, I called her up and asked if she wanted to go with me to the mountains for the weekend. I'm not sure what motivated me to make that call. I'd been dating a woman named Teresa off and on and hadn't seen that much of my future wife who I assumed was still whooping it up at UNC with Tisdale. I think I was bored, and the Lisa scratch still itched. So I made the bold move.

She agreed to go, and the two of us set out for Boone, North Carolina, for a getaway. I loved Grandfather Mountain, not the swinging bridge part, the *real* Grandfather Mountain. To really hike it, you start not on the front touristy side, but on the back side, across the street from a Scotchman grocery and gas station. I had hiked it on numerous occasions with other friends and felt comfortable sharing it with someone I wanted to impress. The view from the top was magnificent. I thought if I took Lisa up there, she'd be impressed with my manly hiking abilities. Being a less macho dude and more of the sensitive type, I prefer Emeril Lagasse to Charles Barkley, I thought this experience might gain me a few cool points. Something I thought I needed to compete with Tisdale.

I think any cool points I accumulated were lost when I decided, at the top of the mountain, to floss my teeth.

I am a nut about gum care. I've never had a cavity and am grossed out by bad teeth. If I meet someone who has plaque buildup, it takes days for me to get the thought of their gooped up teeth out of my mind. I've never ridden the rides at the North Carolina State Fair because so many of the workers have really bad teeth. My theory is that if they can't take care of their mouth, how in the heck can they set up and operate an amusement ride? I am also against riding anything that can be packed up on a truck and transported down I-40. I do not like seeing a Tilt-A-Whirl on the highway.

As I sat on top of the mountain with the woman I secretly loved, looking out on one of the most beautiful scenes in the world, I got an idea. Why not marry the three things that I most loved, all at one time? Why not floss on top of Grandfather Mountain with Lisa? So, I opened my knapsack and pulled out a container of minty fresh, waxed, Johnson & Johnson and went to work. I sort of expected my actions to set our relationship back about seven months. But for those two minutes, life was good.

Surprisingly my actions did not bother Lisa; she laughed and rolled her eyes. That eye roll became a hallmark of our relationship. Me doing something stupid, half out of seriousness and half for the laugh. Her tilting her head and rolling her eyes in a way that only she could.

That spring I accompanied Lisa to her Senior Formal for the Alpha Delta Pi Sorority at UNC. I was five years her senior and was very self-conscious about attending such an event. I drank, a lot, and nearly peed my pants on the bus ride over to the Durham Marriott from the Sorority House on Rosemary Street in Chapel Hill. Once there, the guy checking I.D.'s at the door looked at my driver's license and said, "Stamp him twice." *Bastard.*

After this weekend, Lisa and I began to spend a fair amount of time together. I was a bit older and sort of knew how to make inroads with the players who would be influencing Lisa's decisions. I was also fairly strategic.

During exams, I baked a large batch of brownies and delivered them to the ADPi house just when I knew she and her three roommates were at the peak of studying. What a welcome break: a charming man, a big old pan of brownie and a gallon of milk. I really liked her girlfriends, and it was my intent for them to like me too. I didn't need them planting negative seeds in Lisa's head about the icky old guy from Raleigh who had a crush on her.

In addition to her friends, I needed an in with the family. At some point that spring, Lisa spent a few days at her grandparent's house in Raleigh. She'd been sick and crashed there for the weekend. She was very close to Tutu and Papa, she talked about her grandmother with great affection. They were the grandparents who lived in the same town, the ones who filled in when mom and dad weren't around.

I knew Tutu was larger than life, a big personality, much like her granddaughter who I was falling in love with. When I dropped by their house with a Tupperware container full of freshly-picked strawberries and a bowl of confectioners' sugar, Tutu was impressed. From that moment on, her grandmother referred to me as Mr. Wonderful, a title I proudly wore until her death in 2007.

Chapter 7

1995

My brother's wife told me that her mother, Margaret, worked with a woman at the NC Justice Department who was very, very difficult to get along with. Margaret said she tried to like the woman, she tried hard. However, the woman was just difficult and unkind.

One day Margaret was at the cemetery putting flowers on her grandmother's grave, and she saw the unlikeable woman on her hands and knees tending two grave-stones. When the woman left, Margaret walked over and realized that both the woman's son and husband had died. Margaret suddenly had a deeper understanding of why she might have lost some of her gentleness.

Living with the pressure of disease, in particular a serious condition that could end with death, is inconceivable, even when you are going through it. It is impossible to concentrate on anything except the condition of the patient, the possible outcomes, the future. Interestingly, the future is both your biggest concern and is almost fully taken from you all at the same time.

Prior to cancer, I had a vivid image of what my life would be. I remember one day, before Lisa and I had children, sitting at the base of our staircase waiting for Lisa to get dressed. We were going out to dinner, just the two of us. I had a beer in hand and was listening to Eric Clapton on the stereo. When "You Look Wonderful Tonight" came on, I literally wept. I had never felt such contentment in my life. Lisa and

I were having a conversation — she at the top of the staircase in our bedroom finishing up whatever women finish up the last 30 minutes before a date. Me, ready to go but as happy as could be waiting for the woman I loved to come out of that room, anticipating what to me was the most beautiful woman in the world.

I could imagine children, girls of course. I was a "girl guy" I'd been told, and I knew I'd be extremely content with a house full of women. I wanted four. My argument for four stemmed around family trips to amusement parks. With four children, everyone would have someone to ride with. With one or three, someone would be left out. And who would that be? Invariably, the dad. I do not like to ride rides by myself. I do not like to do anything by myself; thus the need for four kids, all girls. They would all resemble their mother. They would all be strong like their mother. They'd all be a heck of a lot of fun, like their father.

Lisa said I was full of crap — that we couldn't afford four kids and we certainly weren't adding extras for a once in every ten year trip to an amusement park. She agreed to ride alone which appeased me for the moment.

I think I amused her throughout her life. But it must have been tiring to live with someone who constantly had cockamamie ideas. Who would insist that you discuss things like birthing four children for the purpose of amusement park trips? She used to go to YMCA conferences early in our marriage when we both worked there. I would be the keynote speaker on a subject like leadership. After my presentation, people would come up to her and say, "Your husband is so funny." In a monotone voice she would reply, "You should live with him."

I envisioned girls growing up, Lisa giving them their wings and independence, me giving them the nurture. I knew I would struggle letting go; I struggled to let go of my parents, but Lisa would be there, and she was capable of pushing them just enough. We'd be an incredible duo.

I envisioned the years with no children in the house. How difficult it would be when they all left but how much fun it would be to have her all to myself again. We'd get season tickets to the theatre, to NC State and UNC games, the symphony. We'd eat out every night and go see movies. There would be great romance. We'd have enough money to buy about anything we'd want. Life would be perfect.

For 20 years I thought about retirement daily. I wasn't sure what I'd do all day if I retired, but I sure as heck thought I'd like to find out. I could imagine Lisa and me at the beach full time, building fires late at night in an outdoor pit while sipping red wine.

I knew I'd die first. I was male and five years her senior. She'd be with me as I passed on to heaven, holding my hand, softly weeping, glad I wouldn't have to suffer any longer. She'd be so old there'd be no need to remarry. Besides, how could she find anyone as much fun as me?

I could almost put dates by the events in my future, including the social, family and career aspects of my life. And it was good. It was a good, good life.

Now it was difficult to see past next week. And the longer it took to get the answers about her disease, the dimmer our future seemed.

I don't think that the average person can imagine the agony that many people carry. We proceed through life, concerned about the minutiae — a disagreement with our supervisor, a child who makes a C, a mother-in-law who is nosey. None are important.

I did the same, until September 2009.

Chapter 8

1992 – 1993

My family says "I love you" a lot. Every time we talk on the phone, we end with "I love you!" followed by an "I love you too." We probably overuse the term. However, there is no doubt in my mind that my parents love me, unconditionally, and will forever.

Lisa's family isn't nearly as gushy as mine. "I love you" is saved for special occasions, not as a substitute for "Goodbye" over the phone. Permars do express their love on a regular basis, they just do it through fun and humor. If you are cracked on, you are loved.

In 2009, the entire Permar clan took a week-long adventure to Yellowstone National Park in Wyoming. We picked up various family members at airports along the way and descended upon Jackson Hole where we quickly packed into our white 16 passenger van.

At some point early in the week, we decided to give each other trip nicknames which stuck with us throughout the vacation. I was "Wood," named after my grandfather, Woodrow. It was strong, unlike "Bruce." Each of the girls got to choose their own names: Annie T. – "Brookie," Lucy – "Pokie," a name Annie made up while reading a book one night, and Bailey – "Lizzy B.", a shortened form of her first name Elisabeth. For some reason, we dubbed Hayes "Duckie" and David "Santa Claus," perhaps because he had white hair and a large belly or perhaps because he was funding the experience. I'm not sure which.

On our previous trip, Sallie's husband Matt actually proposed to her the night before our vacation. As we waited for them in the airport, my father-in-law said, "I thought Mark and Sallie would be here by now." Yes, he called his soon to be son-in-law Matt, Mark. Three years later, we held on to that blunder and Matt became "Mark" for the week. Ann had always liked the name "Eleanor," and we agreed it fit her affinity for a time gone by. Sallie had an infant on this trip and kept telling us to "shush it." She was afraid we were going to wake the baby. Thus, "Shushit" (pronounced in two different ways depending upon our feelings about Sallie at the time) stuck. Lisa became "Virginia." She often joked about naming a daughter Virginia Ham. Now was her chance to put the names together without ongoing lifetime ridicule.

I'm not aware of many families who would take the time to rename each other on vacation. And I'm certainly not sure of many would have stuck to those names throughout the full seven days.

In the spring of 1992, Lisa and I were standing in her parents' driveway leaning on her 1970 light blue Mustang. She was headed back to Chapel Hill. I was headed to my apartment for a night out with my best buddy, Andy. I looked at her and blurted out, "I think I'm falling in love with you."

Her response was, "I know I'm falling in love with you." I had never said that to another girl before. It wasn't that I was unable to express my feelings, it was that I'd never felt that way about anyone until I met Lisa. I can't explain it exactly. I thought about her constantly. I looked forward to being with her. With every other woman I'd dated, given the choice, I'd rather have been going out with Andy to Crowley's Bar than going out on a date. If Andy was busy, sure I'd go out. If he wanted to hit a bar, I knew we'd have more fun than a date with some girl I had scant interest in, trying to make conversation, wishing I was hanging out with my buddies. And a night out with friends was always a lot less expensive.

Because throwing those words out was not something that Lisa did on a regular basis, either, I think I was the only guy that she said "I love you" to — it was a first for both of us.

We got engaged on February 20, 1993. I tried to work out all of the bugs beforehand. I took Lisa's father to lunch to ask for permission to marry his daughter. His response? "Son, you don't know what a burden you're taking off of me." He then stared up to the sky and mumbled, "Her sister is going to be much harder to place." That indeed did ring true.

The night of our engagement, I reserved the window seat at Est Est Est, which at the time was a nice restaurant in downtown Raleigh. I was convinced that this was a surprise, working hard to cover my tracks over the weeks I spent waiting for the ring to arrive. To my dismay, there were a couple of hitches I hadn't planned for.

The first hitch occurred when four of our inner-city YMCA boys walked by the window and spotted their two youth counselors sharing a romantic dinner together. It was sort of like seeing your teacher at the grocery store; you really had no idea she ever left the school. These were kids we picked up from low-income neighborhoods on buses and brought back to the Y once a week for a swim/gym program. Yet another thing I loved about Lisa, she learned to drive a bus. She got her Commercial Driver's License, and then drove it into the toughest inner-city neighborhoods in town at night. Absolutely no fear.

Not only did they get to see us out of our shorts and Y T-shirts, but they also knew they would get to deliver the news to all of the Walnut Terrace neighborhood that Bruce and Lisa were on a date. My boss didn't even know we were going out, but these four kids now did.

I finally got up from the table, went outside, gave each boy a high five and told them to get the heck out of my romantic evening.

I didn't realize the second hitch was even a hitch until many years later. Apparently my fiancé to be was so certain that I was going to pop the question that night, that when I went to the bathroom, she stuck her hand in my coat pocket and discovered the small box. She later fessed up to this indiscretion — only after many years of marriage. I believe she told me she just had to be certain that this was indeed going to happen. It's a good thing there was a ring in that box, and that it was for her.

Finally, with my desire to do something a bit out of the ordinary, I'd decided that we would walk from the restaurant to the State Capitol, a few blocks away, where I would pop the question. It was a beautiful historic building in the town where she'd grown up. I thought it a fitting and convenient place to seal the deal.

I'm not sure why it didn't dawn on me earlier, but it was really very cold at night in Raleigh in mid-February. After dinner I asked her if she wanted to take a walk over to the capital and she said, "Are you crazy? It's freezing out there." Now, if you knew you were getting a ring on your finger that night, don't you think you would have gone along with whatever plan the guy carved out? Apparently Lisa's comfort was more important than her desire to be engaged. So we drove the three blocks over to the Capitol where I convinced her to get out of the car and walk up to the steps with me. We parked on the north side of the building. It was too cold to walk to the front so I proposed to her on the steps nearest our car. I should have thought this through. I should have waited until April.

She quickly said "yes," and we immediately drove to her parent's house where her sister and ten of Sallie's best friends, along with her brother and parents were waiting for us. Sallie cried. We went through all of the details. We called my parents and repeated the night's events. After about an hour of elation, I began to get light-headed and nauseated. I thought I was going to pass out. I was overwhelmed. I had made a commitment on that night that I would be bound to for the rest of my life. Oh, I loved her, but marriage? I was scared to death.

I finally told Lisa we had to leave, immediately. When we got back to my place, just the two of us, I remembered why I had made this incredibly bold move. It was quite simple: I was madly in love with her.

Chapter 9

September 29, 2009

I missed a significant amount of school in my day primarily due to insecurities. I had a stomach ache every third day, and it often was a result of something that happened at school the previous day. If anyone looked at me funny, I cowered. I embarrassed easily.

I remember one rainy morning as my mother prepared to take me to school, she noticed a girl walking near the woods at the end of our backyard. I recognized her as Dani Fermage. She lived in an old wooden house down an old dirt road. She had virtually nothing. Her clothes were clearly old and frayed. It was pouring down buckets that day, and my mother wasn't about to let Dani walk the remaining half mile to school. Mom headed to the sliding glass door as she asked me if I knew that girl. I said, "YES! It's Danni Fermage, what in the heck are you doing?" My mom, the wife of a Baptist minister, said, "We're giving that girl a ride to school today." I said, "NO! I'll walk!" My mother said, "Better get your rain boots."

At the time I found it a blessing that Dani refused to ride with us explaining that her mother wouldn't let her get in a car with strangers. She did, however, accept my mother's umbrella. To this day, I can't get over how my insecurities could allow me to be so mean to another human being, especially since I myself had been the target of bullying at times in my childhood. An incident like that, being dropped off at school with Dani, would have caused a three-day stomach ache, enough time for all to forget my humiliation.

When I am sick or have an ailment, I need and want some extra attention. If my knee hurt, I would mention it until Lisa would stop what she was doing and ask me for details. I would assume it was cancer or the HIV virus and would begin planning for an extended hospital stay and the specific details of my funeral.

At this point in life, the fact that I had found a few spots of blood on my toilet paper was about to push me over the edge. My wife had colon cancer, so I couldn't make a big deal about three drops of blood on the TP. And yet, what if ironically, we both had the same thing? Maybe it was something in our water.

I decided to go to my doctor the week after Lisa was diagnosed to talk with him about my inability to sleep. I also knew I'd be able to bring up the blood issue. Lisa was in support of me getting a colonoscopy if for no other reason to get me to shut up about it. Everyone in the family knew that I was VERY regular in my bowel habits. The issue was clearly an over-wiping problem, but in my hypochondriac world, you could never be too safe. When I mentioned it to the doctor, he quickly agreed that I should have the procedure if only for peace of mind. It was mid-September and my insurance changed on October 1, which would have increased the cost of the procedure from a $70 co-pay to a couple of thousand dollars bill. Although I get concerned about my health, the overriding factor of following up on medical care for me is the cost. I am cheaper than I am paranoid. So I set the appointment for September 30 before my insurance change.

Journal Entry 9-29-09

*Have my colonoscopy tomorrow. A dot of blood on my t-paper. A bit scary when your wife has just been diagnosed with colon cancer. Haven't eaten all day. Hungry as hell—could **eat** my colon.*

Journal Entry 9-30-09

I have pooped for 24 hours nonstop. Had my colonoscopy today and all was clear! <u>Butt </u>you drink this thick salt water and then poop like you're getting paid for it. I went from 7 pm –1 am, at 5:45 am and from 8 am–3:30 pm. And you couldn't eat for about 48 hours prior to the procedure. It was water by the end — so pure you could have drunk what came out. Lost 8 lbs!

If the shoe had been on the other foot, if I had been diagnosed with cancer, I don't think Lisa would have been so self-centered. I was freaking out about *my* health. I was concerned about what the potential of life without her would mean for *me*. I don't think this behavior was new — in many ways I'd always been somewhat self-absorbed. Our family's cancer situation just magnified it.

Chapter 10

Fall 1993

Being the son of a Baptist minister, I attended a LOT of weddings in my young life. However, I don't think I attended a wedding with a reception outside of the church until I was in college. Snyder Memorial Baptist Church had a large and beautiful sanctuary, and an ample Fellowship Hall. And that's where you held your reception. With no alcohol.

I've seen punch of every color. Punch with lime sherbet, ginger ale, cool whip, and ice rings. I've seen punch dipped out with a ladle and punch flowing from various orifices in the punch bowl structure. I've seen single spewers and multi-layer spewers. Yes, I've had some punch in my life.

When we became engaged, I quickly learned that our wedding reception was not going to be in the church Fellowship Hall. We were going to party at the Cardinal Club, a swanky private dinner club on the 28th floor of the second tallest building in downtown Raleigh. I knew my mother-in-law had impeccable taste and would plan the perfect reception. Every "i" would be dotted, and every "t" would be crossed. Although I knew she would pay attention to the details, I was still surprised when two months before our November wedding in 1993, Ann visited the club to test the tortellini. Yes, she tested the tortellini. No, she didn't taste it; she tested it. My very refined mother-in-law began to fret that the pasta might slide off the plate when you ate it — that it would be difficult to fork. So she called the chef and had him cook up a pot, and she proceeded to head over to test it. With the plates and forks we would be using that night, she stabbed the dish in multiple directions to insure that the little boogers didn't slide. And thank God that she did. Can you imagine attending a reception, dressed in your favorite outfit with tortellini flying all over the room? Oops, that one landed on my shoe. Damn, hit the preacher in the eye. Another one in Mrs. Stamey's cleavage. It could have been disastrous.

Thankfully, the pasta passed the forking test and tasted delicious with the other cuisine served that night.

We had a big affair, 600 people in attendance. At one point before the wedding my father-in-law told me he would give me $10,000 to elope. Ann said, "Hold out for more." And she was right, by a long shot I imagine.

In August of that year, Lisa was at work planning the Y basketball schedule for the season. Our secretary said something about not holding ball games on Nov. 20 because of the annual Raleigh Christmas Parade. Lisa said, "And, it's my wedding day!" She paused and repeated herself, "It is my wedding day, and my church is on the corner of Morgan and Hillsborough Streets, the main route of the parade!" And the wedding was scheduled for 11 am — about the time seven high school marching bands would be belting out *Jingle Bells* with a pounding percussion outside of the sanctuary windows.

Invitations had been ordered but fortunately not yet printed. It took about two weeks for Lisa and her mother to agree upon a new time for the wedding. Her mother was pushing for afternoon and Lisa and I wanted a nighttime event.

Ann suddenly developed grave concern about all of the older people from Fayetteville, my hometown, driving 60 miles in the dark to the wedding. I wasn't sure anyone south of Raleigh over the age of 50, with the exception of my parents, was invited. Lisa and I did not share her concern.

I assured my fiancé, "These people are from a military town. They're tough! Fake bombs are dropping all around them every day. They can handle I-95 after 9 pm!"

I'm not sure why we were so stuck on a late wedding. I thought it sort of seemed more party-esque. Maybe it made Lisa feel more like Cinderella.

I had become so concerned that they wouldn't agree on a time that I called Lisa's dad to ask him what we should do. "*We* do nothing," he emphatically instructed me. "Stay out of it!" It was one of the best pieces of advice my father-in-law has ever given me. I've found it useful in numerous situations throughout my life.

After much discussion, Lisa's mom called one afternoon, "6:30?"

"I like it."

"Meet me at the florist at 4."

Lisa grabbed her jacket and yelled back at me, "The wedding will be at 6:30."

"Huh?"

"6:30. Going to firm up the flowers with Mom."

It was like a mafia deal. I had no idea what had just happened. With no warning or white flag, a compromise was found and business was carrying on as usual.

I didn't realize it at the time, but later in life I'd need to execute the same sort of transactions with my girls. It was good for me to see the mother/daughter relationship so seamlessly at work.

My father married us at First Presbyterian Church on Saturday, November 20, at 6:30 pm. It was beautiful, and we danced the night away at the Cardinal Club after the service. We lined up Tutu and Papa to drive us to a hotel near the airport immediately after the reception. I had booked what I thought would be an amazing honeymoon to the remote island of St. Bart's in the French West Indies. As we walked toward the elevator to head down for the throwing of the rice, an older gentleman who was a longtime friend of Lisa's grandparents, handed me a key. I looked at him puzzled, "What's this for?"

"You may not remember, but I am retired from American Airlines."

"Yea."

"I've got bad news. You aren't going on your honeymoon. All the pilots have gone on strike. I got the call about 7."

"Seriously?"

"Yea. Seriously. This key will open up my beach house in Wilmington. Use it if you like. I don't think you're gonna make it to the Caribbean."

He was right, and as disappointed as we were, we enjoyed a relaxing week on the North Carolina coast, and we were able to rebook our trip for the spring.

We were ecstatic to be with each other, ready to begin a long, happy life together. And to our knowledge, no one was injured by flying tortellini at the Permar-Ham reception.

Chapter 11

September 2009

Email 9-11-09
To: Lisa
From: Bruce

I thought someone emailed you yesterday with an appointment next week at Duke. Is that correct? Trying to get it on my calendar.
B

Response from Lisa:

Just got off the phone with 2 people at Duke. I'm very popular and everyone wants to see me—
Tuesday 9/15—putting in a port—need a driver—7 am bloodwork at the Duke Clinic followed by 8:30 am Duke North procedure to put the port in—involves anesthesia—I would say it will take at least till lunchtime. L

My wife was one of only a few who thought she was popular because numerous cancer schedulers were contacting her about coming to the hospital for various procedures.

We headed to Duke on September 15 for the port surgery. A port is a device they insert under the skin on the chest. You can actually see it poke out not far from the right shoulder. It's like a small pin cushion. From what I can tell, they give you the port under the guise that you won't get poked as much in your veins, "We can draw blood from the port, give you chemo through the port, give you transfusions through the port, heck, we can even feed you oatmeal through the port."

The nurse then inserts one needle into your port and all other sticks go into IV lines connected to the initial needle. This system is meant to replace constant pricks in your arm and hand veins. The needle in the port can stay in for a week or two without being changed.

It sounds like a real time-saver, but in reality half of the nurses in any given hospital aren't trained in how to access the port IV lines. Lisa, being strong-willed, spent many a day at Duke arguing with staff members who did not want to use her port.

"Why did I get a port if you aren't going to use it?" she'd say in a firm, yet kind, manner.

"Well, I'm not trained for that," the new technician would tell her.

"Then you go find someone who is."

I didn't blame her. I hate needles. She had a frickin' rubber dartboard in her chest and yet they still wanted to dig into her veins with a huge syringe.

Lisa emailed a friend about this procedure two days after surgery.

Email, 9-17-09

No one told me that "port insertion" was really "shoulder surgery"—I can't lift my arm to take my shirt off so I'm stuck in my PJs — plus I can't drive or shower today — again, something they didn't tell me until I was doped up on anesthesia. And later

Bruce, who can't stand the sight of blood, has to come home to change my dressings. Should be fun . . .
 Lisa

I did have to change the dressing on her port incision. And I was proud and boasted about it to anyone who would listen. Two weeks after being diagnosed, Lisa was becoming a warrior against cancer, and I was becoming Florence Nightingale. I was amazed at what I could do when it came down to it. I learned that I could nag, "Lisa, it's time to change the dressing."

"Not now."

"Yes now. It's been 12 hours and we're changing it. Now. Unbutton your shirt."

Except for "unbutton your shirt," none of the other words in that exchange had ever come out of my mouth. I didn't remind people to do stuff; people reminded me. I didn't clean out incisions or cuts or scrapes, I hated blood. Lisa was in charge of all boo boos.

Not anymore. I was getting fairly cocky. I suggested that I could have actually done the surgery for the port. No response was given from the patient.

On September 16, Sallie was in town and took Lisa to Duke to be measured for radiation. The radiology doctor told them that although they could not confirm it, they all were confident that the ovary was malignant. There you go, a Mike Tyson stomach punch again.

I continued to be surprised that as much as we knew the answers to the difficult questions before we went in to the doctor's office, hearing the news directly from their mouth was devastating. It almost made me physically ill. With each new hit of bad news, I would be mentally setback for days.

With each setback, I talked. The way I deal with life is to talk it out. Over and over and over again. My mother was one of the people I confided in.

Journal: 9-19-09

Mom thinks I'm grieving for something that probably won't happen. Although I do have some thoughts around "what if" and it scares and saddens me, I think I'm perhaps more grieving over the loss of life BC (before cancer). I think about our summer: vacations, laughter, family time without worry, sex and excitement around courting my wife. All are still possible, all come out now in glimpses, but all happiness, right now, quickly becomes overshadowed by CANCER. It's everywhere...on the voice mail, e-mail, text – grocery store, meals arriving at the door, visitors and house guests that wouldn't be here without it. The dread of another trip to Durham where you might find out more...the worry for your kids and constant art Annie T. produces all designed to make mom better. Knowing that for the rest of Lisa's life we'll, or at least I, will be looking over my shoulder for IT to creep up on us again. We'll beat it this time, I think we will.

Lisa had a wonderful group of girlfriends from high school. There were five of them: Kim, Francie, Susan, Charlotte and Lisa. We were the only ones who still lived in Raleigh. Being in their hometown, the other classmates dropped by on occasion when visiting family or friends.

All of these women were strong. All cared deeply about each other.

I was closest to Charlotte. She worked with me at the YMCA when she was in high school and college and had coached me through my relationship with Lisa. She was not married, although she has dated most men in the United States. Although all of these women, Lisa included, would speak their mind, Charlotte had no qualms about calling me out when needed.

Two weeks after we found out Lisa had cancer, this group of women were scheduled to take their annual trip, this time to Boulder, Colorado, Charlotte's home. Lisa just wasn't up to traveling a long distance after coming off of surgery for her port so they all decided to come to North Carolina and whisk her away to the mountains for the weekend.

This was great for all of them but very tough for me. It gave me an entire weekend to stew, something I've always been very good at.

Journal Entry, September 23, 2009

Charlotte left at 5 am Monday morning. I drove her to the airport. When she was leaving, she said that I had to get myself together. She said Lisa needs not to worry about me. She said it is natural for her to worry some about me but that I need to do all I can to keep her from carrying my load. She said on Thursday when we were told that they strongly suspected that there was cancer in her ovary I looked like I'd been hit by a truck. She said I had to do better. She was adamant that I had to develop a more positive outlook and quick. I'm not sure that's possible.

Different people take on different roles as you move through an illness. Charlotte's role was to kick me in the ass. Others prepared food, or wrote notes — the mailbox was full for a solid nine months. Many were prayer warriors. They didn't do a very good job.

Journal Entry September 23, 2009 (cont'd)

Today I was working out at the Y doing my regular weight room routine when I spotted a friend and Y board member, Holly. She is an encourager and has the faith of Moses. After a brief update, she asked if we could pray. I said sure. She grabbed my hands and we stood, arm in arm, together in the middle of the Y workout room. Her words were strong. Her prayer was passionate. She asked God to give me a "battle shield." I'm not sure I know exactly what that looks like and I'm not convinced I'm strong enough to carry it. It sounded quite large and very heavy.

Today and yesterday have been better emotionally. We were to start treatment tomorrow but all was cancelled due to some screw up with the ovarian pathology report. All has been pushed back to next week. So, we sit, waiting to proceed. Surgery first or treatment? Colon cancer? Ovarian cancer? Lisa gets emotionally ready to move forward, we get all logistics covered — work, carpools for the kids — and we're ready to move. We don't want it to spread any more. It seems that every minute we wait another major organ develops a new tumor. Oops, we made a mistake on your pathology report—we'll call back next week. It's not like they forgot to leave tomatoes off our burger! It's MY WIFE'S LIFE that's at stake here! No room for mistakes! Get the frickin' order right!

Journal Entry, September 25, 2009

Earlier in the week I had a great conversation with Brad's [my best friend] sister who is a GI Oncological nurse at Baptist Hospital in Winston. She talked about the new drugs out to battle GI cancers. She said one that Lisa will be taking is a miracle drug. She was concerned that they were not doing a biopsy on the ovary — I think that's a good question. She said she has stage 4 patients with survival rates of 5, 7, 8 years — What about 9, 10, 11??? What did that mean?? Is the year 8 person still alive? Is 8 the max?? So I start thinking about 8 years from now — Bailey 20, Lucy Powell 17, Annie T. 14 — my boss retiring — oh, the places my mind goes —

Chapter 12

1993 – 1994

Before Lisa and I were married, I decided to move out of my small apartment and buy a 1,000 square foot house that was built in 1918. The house was in Five Points, an old Raleigh neighborhood that was coming back to life. It was a gray bungalow with intricate wooden shingles on the front face of the house. The front door had a big glass window and a mail slot. That freaked me out a bit. What would keep someone from putting a snake through the slot? Or a scorpion?

When my brother, Chad, got married the first time, I was merciless. I was 18 years old and was beside myself at the thought of being a best man. I devised all sorts of ways to torture him on his wedding day. First, I sewed his tuxedo pant legs together with a needle and some white thread. He got his pants half way on, and I heard a scream, "Mom! Something's wrong with these pants!" Chuckling, I opened his suitcase and sewed each pair of his underwear together where your legs poke out. As if that wasn't enough, I filled each of his socks with shaving cream. My brother had known me a very long time; I was a bit surprised that he was so lackadaisical about his belongings that day.

When we got to the church, I worked with a good friend of the family, Lamar Clark, a man my parents' age, to condomize anything in his car we could find — the gear shift, radio knobs, antenna, door handles – and with spermicide. You just can't be too safe.

And to top it off, Mr. Clark showed me how to take the sardines I had purchased, and put them in the engine where the heat from the car would blow into the air conditioning unit. Perhaps I was the root cause of their divorce 14 years later. After my antics, I'm not sure my sister-in-law ever really felt accepted by me. Looking back on it, I can sort of see why.

A decade later, when I got married, Chad and his wife remembered what I had done. Unfortunately for them, they were old. They had two kids and simply didn't have the energy to repay my youthful antics. The only thing they could think of to get me back was to stuff my infant niece's stinky diaper in the mail slot where it sat for seven days until Lisa and I returned from our honeymoon.

The house was cute but small. When I purchased it, I thought I had purchased two bedrooms with two closets. On the day I moved in, I began putting stuff in one of the closets. When I finished unpacking that room, I went to the closet in the other room. Upon opening the door, I realized that I had entered the same closet I had just left. I felt duped, although I guess it was my responsibility to really dig through the house before purchasing.

The back of the house had a slanted roof which added a great deal of charm. It also added a kink in your neck if you peed standing up. The one toilet was on the very back wall of the house. If you stood for number one, you had to lean back or your face would press against the angled ceiling. It's amazing that I don't have brain damage as many times as I went to the bathroom at night during my two years on Sunrise Avenue. People at work thought I had a birthmark on my forehead. It was an ongoing bruise.

I wasn't sure what to expect with marriage. I loved my new wife, and she seemed fairly easy to get along with. We liked many of the same things, so I figured this would be an easy transition. In most regards it was. In a few, it was not.

One area where we struggled to see eye-to-eye was with our finances. It didn't take long to discover that we did not manage our money in the same fashion. I was prudent with my purchases and balanced my checkbook to the penny. If I had less than $1,000 in my checking account, from my perspective, I was broke. If I saw a shirt that I liked, regardless of the cost, I would walk away and ponder the purchase for a day, a week, a month.

Lisa on the other hand enjoyed spending. If she went to the ATM and it reported she had $1,242 in her account, it was hers to spend. It did not matter that she had three outstanding checks that had not yet cleared the bank. It did not matter that the phone bill was due on Tuesday. She had $1,242 available bucks at that moment in time, and she wasn't going to let it go to waste.

Because my parents had always shared everything and because my mother did not work much outside of the house, they had one checking account. I assumed we would too. Not so. Lisa told me that she was keeping her own checking account. Her argument? "If I need to go to Belk and spend $60 on hose, and you can easily do that you know (I didn't), I don't need you asking me why I went to Belk and spent $60 on hose. I work. I make money. I'll have my own checkbook." It sort of hurt my feelings that she did not want me to fix her financial situation. In my view, it was in shambles. She didn't have any debt, but she didn't have any assets either — unless you count the hose.

Over the years, we grew comfortable with me covering all of the bills and her covering all of the extemporaneous expenses. I grew less concerned with balancing to the penny, it simply took too damn long and really, what was the point? She grew more concerned with savings and bigger purchases and once even tried to balance her checkbook.

I don't think Lisa ever knew how much money she had. She always had enough to pay off her credit card each month, and she saved money for retirement and to pay for all of the kids' big ticket items like resident camp, piano and dance. I think she just had a sixth sense as to when she had to hold off on purchasing until her next paycheck arrived.

In addition to learning how to come to terms with differences in our handling of finances, we found other areas where we were going to need to compromise to live in wedded bliss.

My wife was a very accomplished woman. She tackled life with a zest that few people possess. Lisa chaired committees at the Junior League. She led children's choir at church and put together a musical for 50 kids. Lisa wrote the long-range plan at our church and spearheaded the effort that raised $3,000,000 for our children's small private school's capital campaign. But on Saturday, she sat; often for hours on end.

There is a TV channel that shows back-to-back reruns of the 80's drama *90210*. Lisa could sit and watch four or five of those shows in a row. Read the paper, watch an episode. Eat some breakfast, watch another episode. Sit up, watch another episode.

I, on the other hand, got up on Saturdays and made a comprehensive list of all the things I wanted to accomplish.

Make a list
Eat breakfast
Wash, dry, fold and put up dark clothes
Wash, dry, fold and put up white clothes
Clean the toilet
Clean the sink
Clean the shower
Vacuum
Dust
Mow
Edge
Blow
Buy flowers
Plant flowers
Exercise
Grocery store

Because I liked to mark things off the list, it gave me a sense of accomplishment, I included things like "Make a List" –- a quick, easy win for the morning.

I would share the list of things that needed to get done with Lisa, and she would watch another episode. I would leave the list on the kitchen counter with a marker, intended to encourage someone to do something on the list and cross it off; she would watch another episode. And as she read the paper or talked on the phone or watched TV, I would get madder and madder and madder. After I cleaned the toilet, I would work to express my frustration by slamming the toilet lid down as hard as I possibly could. Lisa would turn up the volume.

After about two years of marriage and a huge elephant in the room between us, I mustered up the courage to announce my displeasure.

"I am frustrated. I have a very long list that needs to be accomplished, and I need your help. I do ALL of the work around here on the weekends – YOU watch TV. Help me!"

Lisa came back strong, "I too am frustrated. I do not like a Saturday list. I work hard during the week and need down time on the weekend. I do not intend to spend my day vacuuming a rug that is not dirty. If I spill something on it, I'll clean it up. Stop trying to plan my day for me. Why can't you sit still and just spend some time with me?"

I simply didn't understand that some people needed time to sit and veg. I didn't need that – I needed to complete the list.

Finally, after a few years of pent up frustration with each other, Lisa said, "Why don't we get a maid? If we are both going to work full-time, let's invest in some help with the house."

And at that moment, we stopped trying to change each other. We got help which lightened my load and relieved her sense of guilt. And I learned to be a little less uptight and to relax a little with my wife. We were getting the hang of this marriage thing.

Chapter 13

October 1, 2009

The first day of treatment was quite an education for Lisa and me. She had been measured for radiation, but it took a very long time to get her positioned precisely to receive treatment. Every millimeter counted. The radiation had to go in at the exact right place, and it had to be precise for each of the daily treatments — 30 of them.

I'm not 100% sure what they did to Lisa in the treatment room, but she did share that it was humiliating — especially initially. She lay on a hard table with nothing on below the waist. The radiation beam was shot into specific spots. If she moved one bit, they would have to reposition her. It was emotionally and physically exhausting.

In addition to the radiation, Lisa's treatment included a continuous chemotherapy IV drip through her port. The chemo was in an IV bag inserted into a fanny pack that Lisa wore for the entire six weeks of radiation.

As if all of the medical issues weren't enough, she now had to contend with a fanny pack.

This might not have been an issue for some women. There are actually people who choose to wear these comfortable and handy butt pouches, but not my wife. Lisa had impeccable style. Like me, she was somewhat of a clothes horse — often purchased on sale, but from the nicest stores in town. Her fanny had never seen a pack before, and she was not happy about this one.

The following week her best girlfriends met her for lunch. All four of them donned a fanny pack in a gesture of solidarity! They laughed and laughed and took pictures. In Lisa's mind, they had made a significant sacrifice: entering a trendy Midtown restaurant willingly wearing a dorky fanny pack. One even had Mickey Mouse on it.

As usual, Lisa was a good sport and did not complain once on this crazy marathon day. After radiation, we checked in at Chemo Central and then grabbed a bite to eat. Apparently they don't mix your drugs until you arrive at the clinic. Unlike ketchup, its half-life is short.

When we were finally called back to the Drip Room, I nearly passed out. It was dark with a low ceiling and florescent lights. It was sterile and stark. There were blue, pleather recliners that lined the walls. There were other smaller chairs arranged throughout the large room — back-to-back, side-by-side; no space was left unused. The nurse who took Lisa's vitals struck up a conversation. I was working diligently to act as if this was no different than a trip to McDonald's.

"Hey baby, how you doing?" she said to Lisa.

"I'm alright, but I think my husband's about to pass out."

"Honey, you'd be surprised how many of them we lose in here. Just the other day a man dropped right here by this chair. Thank God we're the ones who have the babies."

I interjected: "In my defense, I am in a room with more needles than a church has Bibles. Until now I had not mentioned that fact, and I do not even feel lightheaded. Do you want me to access her port?"

"Baby, you talk a big game!"

Our chemo nurse, Fran, was nice but awkward. She talked to herself throughout the process of inserting the needle into Lisa's chest. At times I thought she was talking to me, and it did not give me confidence.

"Let's see, gotta get this untangled here."

"Untangled, what's tangled?"

"Oh this tube. It's fine. Now what size needle do I need?" she said as she thumbed through a drawer as if she was going to experiment until she discovered the one that worked best.

"You're skinny. Earlier today I had to access a port and the woman had the biggest boobs you've ever seen in...your...life. I thought I'd never get it in there. You're gonna be a piece of cake."

After Fran pulled out all of the equipment, Lisa noticed her new appendage, a burgundy fanny pack. Being the top notch dresser that she was, she immediately honed in on the color.

"Fran, do the fanny packs come in black? I don't wear any burgundy."

Fran and I exchanged a glance — I'm sure she was thinking the same thing I was: *You have stage 4 colon cancer. This bag carries poison that will be injected into your system through a needle that is about to be inserted in your chest. And you're concerned about the color of the fanny pack?*

I didn't realize it at the time, but after spending seven weeks with Fran, I figured out why this question seemed even the odder to her. From what I could tell, she only owned one shirt. It had a scene from a city in Europe. At week four I commented to Lisa, "Back in Paris!" She informed me that Fran actually had two shirts, but that they were difficult to distinguish. One was Paris; one was Rome.

Fran politely looked at Lisa, "Well, I don't think I've been asked that question before, but if it will make you happy, I'll go look."

"Thank you."

Fran scooted away.

I looked at Lisa, "Really?"

"I don't have any burgundy clothes! It's bad enough that I have to wear this damn thing. The least they can do is give me one that's neutral."

Thankfully Fran returned with a black fanny pack. Lisa's level of stress seemed to immediately diminish.

"Thank you."

Lisa squeezed my hand as Fran inserted the first needle into what would become the main highway for foreign matter to enter into her bloodstream. I was glad she squeezed — I felt so useless.

After the chemo began, we had to sit there for several hours to insure that it wouldn't immediately kill her. Fran talked us through how to change the chemo bags, read the messages from the chemo pump and showed us how to replace the batteries. I took notes furiously, fearing that I'd be the one who would need to act if something went wrong. As usual, until Lisa was on significant pain meds much later in her illness, she handled all alarms and chemo crises on her own. My wife was independent and other than wanting me there for moral support, she was just fine taking care of herself, thank you. In fact, she drove herself to radiation on most days despite countless offers from friends to chauffer.

Journal Entry 10-1-09

First day of treatment. Met with the oncologist, accessed her port for the first time, waited forever for her drugs to be ready. Wow, we just entered the room where there are multiple recliners with cancer patients receiving their chemo IVs. It is truly troublesome. Medical equipment all around, IVs, needles, 5 FU drugs—I need a shower... at least the floors are shiny. How do you work in a place like that? Depressing. These people are compassionate, caring angels sent here to minister to folks – folks who are going through pure hell I'm sure. I feel like I've entered Gray's Anatomy or the set of ER. Never seen anything like it. Keep my eyes on the page—don't look up—might see someone get stuck; someone in pain—emotionally or physically. Old man here alone—how does this happen? Where does cancer come from? At least Ellen's on TV.

The chemo is called 5FU. There is something very fitting about that name. Five &@#* You – &@#* YOU cancer. &@#* you five times or more! &@#* YOU.

Chapter 14

1997 – 2002

I don't specifically recall being told that we were expecting our first child. Perhaps it was in September, just a pregnancy kit at home. I do recall an overwhelming feeling of responsibility. I enjoyed the process of trying to get pregnant so the news in fairly short order was a bit of a letdown.

We attended Lamaze classes at the hospital closest to our house. There were about 12 couples in the course and all but two took things rather seriously. Lisa and I were in that camp. Our instructor, however, took it all *very* seriously. Her classes were well-planned, and she did not hold back one teeny detail.

One night the instructor had the soon to be fathers sit on the floor and prop back on a pillow. His spouse was then told to sit in his lap and practice breathing. Lisa was struggling to get comfortable.

"What's wrong baby? Why are you wiggling?"

"Your belt buckle is jabbing me in the back."

"Oh. I need to remember not to wear a belt on delivery day."

"No worries baby. This is just a breathing exercise. I don't think I'll be lying in the floor propped up against you when the baby actually comes out!"

"Right."

On the night they showed a video of the C-section, I began to get lightheaded. Before they even began the operation, I excused myself. "I cannot watch this, I think I'm going to pass out," I told my wife.

"Go drink some water or something. You are pathetic."

Lisa and I talked about our birth plan. The instructor told us we needed to make decisions about what we wanted to occur during labor and delivery and write it in a notebook to share with our doctor prior to delivery. She discussed natural childbirth and even suggested that we might want to use a tub or whirlpool during labor.

Who in their right mind would have a baby in a whirlpool? Does the doctor get in there with you? Are we all in our bathing suits? Do you need a snorkel? Perhaps you don't have the baby in it; maybe it is a pre-delivery method or something. Come to think of it, being in water can make one need to go to the bathroom, especially if it's warm. Maybe it's the same phenomenon.

After the first night of class, Lisa looked at me and said, "Our birth plan is to get as many drugs in my system as is humanly possible. I want them the second I walk into the hospital. If we go to the hospital and they say I'm not ready to deliver, we will stay the parking lot. That is our plan. You can write it down if you want."

I fully concurred. I did not want to see my wife moaning and groaning in pain while delivering my baby. It's just all so unnatural.

Lisa also told me that I had three other important jobs during delivery. Job one was to stay up by her head. She told me she did not need me down there checking things out. It was private, between her and her doctor.

I said, "Honey, I thought that area was between you and me."

"It *was* between you and me. Now it is between my doctor and me. I don't need the image in my mind of you having that image in your mind. Stay up by my head."

That was fine with me! I'd seen enough childbirth in Lamaze class to last me a lifetime. I agreed it was probably best not to watch.

The second job I had was to make sure the nurse cleaned off the baby before she slapped her on Lisa's chest.

"When the baby comes out, have them wash it off before they give it to me."

"Why?"

"Because I want a Gerber baby moment, and Gerber babies don't have blood all over them."

I'd seen the commercials. She was right. I didn't even know they'd try to slop a nasty, unclean baby on you. I was glad to have something specific to add to the cause.

"Your final job, and I know this is going to be hard for you, is not to make jokes."

I had no problem with jobs one and two, but no jokes?

When we left the delivery room with our first- born daughter, Bailey, the inside of my mouth was as bloody as a Freddie Krueger horror movie victim. I had bitten my tongue so hard all day to keep from cracking jokes that it was like minced meat.

All three of our deliveries were scheduled. Lisa was gestationally diabetic, and they did not want the babies to get too big, so they induced her right around her due date.

On the day that our first child was being delivered, June 28, 1997, we awoke early and headed over to the hospital, about three miles from our house. I don't remember a ton about the day. I assumed Lisa would have taken the epidural the minute they asked, regardless of her level of pain. Instead, for most of the day she said she could handle it sans medication.

When the anesthesiologist finally did come in, I discovered why they are so rich. The nurse sat Lisa up and had her hunch over with her back exposed and rounded. Once Lisa was in place, a masked woman darted into the room. She said, "I'm going to count to three and then you will feel a slight sting. Are you ready?" Lisa responded in the affirmative. "One, two, three…" She grabbed a piece of medical tape, gently tapped it on her back and disappeared seemingly into the wall.

When I reviewed my hospital bill, the anesthesiologist's portion was $6,000.

Lisa and I had pleasant conversation until the last few hours, but there was not a lot of humor. At one point though I called a friend at work to touch base on a project that needed my attention.

"How's it going? Is Lisa OK?"

"Yes. She's fine. She has dilated 7 inches. It should be soon."

When I got off the phone, Lisa was crying — not tears of pain, but tears of laughter.

"What are you laughing at? What's going on?"

"You said I was dilated 7 inches!"

"That's what the nurse just said."

"Centimeters baby! It's not inches it's centimeters. If I was dilated 7 inches, the baby could walk out."

I didn't think it was that funny. But if it made her happy, I was fine to play along.

Like most women, Lisa was strong throughout the 13 hours of labor. She would talk to the nurse asking for a play-by-play description of what to expect next.

Our first daughter, Bailey, was born at 7:32 pm, at Rex Hospital. They asked me if I wanted to cut the cord — I knew the answer to that. "I have to stay up here. I'm not allowed down there. That's private."

My mother-in-law had read that in some countries the placenta is considered a delicacy and offered to cook it up for our next Thanksgiving dinner; we declined the offer. I didn't think she was serious, but I was uncertain enough to ask the nurse to be sure to dispose of it. I was afraid we'd go over one night and her special "meatloaf" would be less meat and more placenta.

When Bailey came out, the nurse gasped. We thought that something was wrong. Lisa said, "Is she OK?" The nurse said, "Yes, but she's blonde." We both had dark hair. Assuming Bailey is my biological child, that is unusual.

The nurse immediately started to put Bailey on Lisa's chest. Lisa elbowed me. I saw the bloody baby coming at her — I almost fell down on job number two. "STOP!" I shouted. The nurse looked at me bewildered.

"She doesn't want the baby on her until you clean her up a bit. She wants a Gerber baby moment." Lisa and I smiled at the nurse. She sort of furrowed her brow, turned quickly and took Bailey to the other side of the room.

Bailey came out as blue as a Smurf, and her head was in the shape of a dunce cap. She looked like an alien. They put a small baby toboggan on her head to help keep her warm. But it didn't do much good. It barely covered the tip top. Her head was as long as Jafar in the Disney movie *Aladdin*.

I questioned the nurse, "What's wrong with her head, and why is she blue?" "Her color will come," and it did as they started to massage her little body.

"Often the first-born child has a more cone shaped head because they are the first to travel through the mother's birth canal — she is a pioneer — it will even out."

Like Daniel Boone. The birth stuff was very technical.

Due to bed space, we were moved out of the maternity ward that night and were put on the fourth floor. And that's when we visited hell.

As we began the process of getting to know our baby, we discovered that breast feeding was going to be difficult. Actually, difficult might be an understatement. Sallie, who thought her degree in epidemiology made her an expert on lactation, told us that we should breast feed as long as possible. "It helps the baby build up her immune system."

Frankly, I didn't care. It was Lisa's decision. If she wanted to feed the kid naturally, I was in full support. If it was difficult or uncomfortable, I was fine to go with formula.

Because we struggled to get Bailey to settle down or to get her to eat, they sent a lactation nurse to assist.

If you are a lactation nurse, you are all about some natural stuff. This is not a criticism. I enjoy nature too and even once took fish oil to reduce my cholesterol. Some, however, take natural to the extreme. These women, and I've never seen a male lactation nurse, are merciless.

A lactation nurse is taught to make people feel horrible and inadequate if they do not breast feed. I believe they are trained to berate you and spout off all the things that can happen if your baby does not eat breast milk his first six years of life. I heard that a bottle-fed child can develop more allergies, infections and is more likely to join a gang. I've been told that Lisa's brother breast fed for multiple years. Come to think of it, he is very hearty. Seldom gets sick, and he isn't in a gang. Lisa and I decided that when you could ask for milk to go with your cookies, it was time to move to the bottle, or the glass.

We left the hospital after 24 hours; we couldn't take anymore. Because we were moved out of the maternity ward and put on a surgical floor, we were low on the priority list. They were dealing with heart transplants and appendectomies. We simply had a baby — a couple of stitches and lactation issues were not a serious concern.

I remember returning home from the hospital the day after Bailey was born. We had no idea what to do. Lisa's mother spent the night with us just because we were afraid. Bailey was a pretty good sleeper from the get-go, but we did have things to learn.

After about ten or twelve days at home, I was changing our new kid's diaper. I loved wet wipes and used them liberally. But on that day, as I was cleaning my child's bottom, I discovered that we had not done a good job of scouring the area. I found a white sort of cheesy matter exactly where it shouldn't be. I yelled for Lisa. Neither of us knew you had to dig so deep to get the area spic and span. I have an excuse in that I don't have one of those. But you'd think my wife would have known to search a little harder for grime in the region.

Of course, we took her to the doctor to make sure this would not negatively affect her in future years — as a parent you could just envision that you caused your child to be sterile due to your lack of attention within the first week of life. The doctor gave us a strange look, examined our daughter and gave us a clean bill of health. I'm sure he also called his friends to share the story.

There were two times that my wife startled me during the first month or so of Bailey's life. Lisa was always a very modest woman. She changed clothes in the closet and could do so without ever showing an inch of skin. I'm not sure how she did it, but she could remove or put on a bra, undershirt, skirt, underwear, you name it, without getting naked. I have seen her remove a jog bra while wearing a sweat suit and long pants without removing another garment. I, on the other hand, enjoy being naked. I find it freeing.

One day after returning to work, I entered the bedroom where I found my wife walking around with one towel wrapped around her head and another around her waist. And that was all.

I said, "Modubu, gaya lacka hunta butu?" She looked like an African tribal woman from the National Geographic magazine. She flipped me off.

She was so sore from nursing that her modesty was gone. I stared in amazement. She said, "Don't even think about it."

My second encounter with a woman who looked like my wife but clearly was not, was week two when I arrived home from work. I walked in the house and called out with no reply. The car was in the drive and the door was unlocked so I was pretty sure she was there with child. I combed the downstairs, nothing. I then moved upstairs. There sat Lisa, tears flowing down her face, rocking our screaming child.

"How's it going baby?" I innocently inquired.

An outpouring of frustration and exhaustion came from my wife. Bailey had not slept all day. She struggled to eat and at 6 pm, she was still crying.

"I'll take her. Let me give you a break."

A look came across my wife's face that I had never seen before. There was something in her eyes. Through sobs and fierce rocking Lisa said, "No. I'll put her down. I am her mother; she will sleep for me."

I couldn't decide if she was just very determined or if she was going to kill our baby. What I did know was that if I did not get my ass out of that room, I would be taken down too. I backed out slowly and grabbed the phone; my thumb on the 9, just in case. In about an hour Lisa came downstairs and acted as if nothing had happened. I asked if she was OK.

"I'm fine."

I slipped upstairs to check for signs of life. Bailey seemed fine and was asleep. I was left perplexed.

Lisa was an incredible mother to our newborn. She read a book that helped her get Bailey sleeping through the night by six weeks. I remember sometime near that time waking up to Bailey's cry.

Lisa said, "I'm tired."

I said, "Me too."

"Leave her?"

"Uh huh."

The next morning we woke up to get ready for work, and Bailey was quiet.

"SIDS!"

I ran into her room only to find her sound asleep. We had turned a corner. We had mastered sleep.

Our second daughter Lucy Powell was born at Rex Hospital almost exactly three years after Bailey. We had no significant issues with the birth but she was a dark skinned, dark-haired, exotic looking baby. Sort of like Sophia Loren.

About four months after Lucy was born, we had another odd incident with the doctor. Lucy Powell began to smell horrible. She was a HUGE slobberer so we kept a bib on her 24 hours a day. If you held her up over your face, as one is want to do with a baby, her spit would flow right into your mouth.

On multiple occasions, we had noticed that Lucy was quite odiferous. We'd give her a bath, and she'd be fine. But after we put her to bed and picked her back up, the odor returned. It seemed to be coming from her ear or the side of her face.

The smell was like rotten eggs. And we had no idea what could be causing it. We'd clean her and invariably in two or three hours she'd smell bad again.

We took her to the doctor and explained our situation. Our practice had ten pediatricians, and we drew the short straw; the young one with no kids of his own. He was tall with blonde hair; relaxed, moved slowly. And he looked at us as if we'd fallen out of a tree.

"So your daughter smells bad?" he inquired.

I could tell he thought we were idiots.

"This is our second child, *Dr. Spock*," I intentionally started my sentence so that he'd know we weren't rookies. "We have a three-year-old, Bailey, and now we have an infant with a chronic stench. What could it be?"

He began sniffing around our baby as he looked in each orifice.

"I really don't smell anything."

"This is an off hour. She just had a bath. Just wait, it'll be back."

"Exactly where does it smell, Mr. Ham?"

"On her face — often near her ear."

He pulled his scope out again and stretched her ear wide as he peered within. By now Lucy was angry.

"Could Bailey have put something in her ear?"

"Like what?" Lisa asked.

"Like a pea or something?"

We look at each other puzzled.

"Do you see a pea in there?"

"Well, no. But I guess there could be remnants that are rotten in her ear canal."

"So what should we do?"

"Well, could you bring her back when the smell returns?"

A $20 copay, and all you can give us is a return visit? Isn't there a prescription to cure stinky baby syndrome? Some physician you are.

"I guess. And we won't serve any more peas."

We returned home and thoroughly questioned our three-year-old.

"Bailey, did you put anything in Lucy Powell's ear?"

"Nope!"

"Bailey, Did you put a pea in Lucy Powell's ear?"

"Nope!"

"Are you sure?"

"Nope!"

The conversation was going nowhere. We were frustrated and dumbfounded. Could this be some sort of birth deformity that we were destined to live with the rest of our lives? We put Lucy back down for a nap and when we woke her up, the odor was back as strong as ever.

I was determined to figure this out. I sniffed her like a bloodhound searching for a fox. And then, like Einstein and electricity, a light bulb went off.

I climbed into her crib. A six foot tall, 175-pound man in his baby's crib, nose to the mattress. And what I found was that although we had washed the sheet on the mattress fairly often, we had never washed the mattress cover. Because Lucy slobbered so much, the cover smelled awful!

"Lisa! I found it. Victory is ours. Our child is normal. It's we who are nuts."

I worried a bit about my judgment of the doctor, but not enough to call him back to let him know that the mystery was solved. I was still a bit ticked that he didn't find something medical which would have spared me my personal humiliation.

We worked a little harder to get pregnant the third time, which was all right by me. The first two came so quickly. Number three wasn't the same. We tried and tried and tried — for months. I was beginning to think my boys had swum their last meet. Someone told me that drinking orange juice would up your sperm count. I was downing a carton a day.

Then finally, I went home one evening when Lisa had a meeting and on the counter she had left me a yellow sticky note. It read: "You can stop drinking OJ. We still have it!" I was elated. I'd always wanted a big family and adding number three was headed in the right direction.

When time arrived for the delivery of our third daughter, Annie T., the epidural did not take the same as it had with the first two births. Apparently the dosage was greater so Lisa's legs were almost fully out of commission.

She could not feel anything, which was good. But she also could not lift or move her legs at all, which was a problem.

When it came time for her to start pushing, she could not get her legs in the stirrups. The nurse lifted her right leg and told me to lift her left leg.

"I can't," I replied in a matter of fact fashion. I was proud that I had remembered our birthing "plan."

"Bruce, I really need you to lift your wife's leg."

"I'm not allowed to go down there. That's between her and her doctor."

Our nurse looked at my wife in disbelief.

And then a weird and interesting thing happened. Lisa's head spun in a 360-degree circle and she bellowed, "LIFT MY LEG!"

"But honey, you said to stay—"

"LIFT MY LEG!"

Was this a trick? Was she trying to test me to see if I would break rule number one? What should I do? I wondered to myself. *I'm supposed to be up by her head, but she is yelling for me to lift her leg. This is a lose-lose situation.*

It was as if time stopped for several minutes while I weighed my options. I looked at the nurse, I glanced at Lisa. I wasn't certain in my decision, but I had to make a move. I slowly shifted toward her left leg. I lifted it gently into the stirrup. And there right in my view, was the crown of my child's head.

I had never seen anything like it. I wanted to look away but couldn't. It was like a train wreck. The horror, the blood. But I had to watch — my eyes fixed on the action.

"It's time to push, Lisa," the nurse instructed. "This isn't going to take long."

My wife obediently and courageously followed the nurse's orders, and Annie T. began to appear.

The doctor ran into the room — he almost missed the moment. And right there, at Rex Hospital, with my wife's left leg in my hand, the most gruesome and beautiful thing I'd ever seen in my life occurred right before my very eyes.

With tears in my eyes I looked up at Lisa. She was crying too. "Cut the cord, honey. Cut the cord."

I moved beyond Lisa's leg and took the scissors from the nurse's hand. And with the tiniest little soul I'd ever seen lying in the doctor's hand, I detached my daughter from her mother.

Lisa looked at me, "Bring her up here."

I took my daughter from the doctor and put her bloody little body right on Lisa's chest.

Although we never really discussed it, I believe we both knew this would be our last child.

Chapter 15

September, 2009

It was a constant struggle to know what to tell our children about Lisa's cancer. Lisa and I were people who typically held nothing back. We were honest and open—not just about cancer, but about most things in life. Although we'd never dealt with anything of this magnitude, our instinct was to be honest with the kids without ensuing panic. We wanted them to have the information they needed to be able to answer questions and share with friends as they chose. We did not want to have to change the topic of conversation when one of them entered the room. We also didn't want them to obsess about something that we knew very little about.

I remember our first conversation about Lisa's cancer. Bailey wasn't at home but was returning that night from a weekend beach trip. We decided to tell Lucy and Annie T. together.

"Girls, you may have heard us talking in the den this afternoon. And you probably noticed that Mommy and Daddy have been crying. Well, we've been crying because we found out today that mom has cancer."

Annie T. threw in the first and most obvious question. It was the same one I was asking myself but wasn't bold enough to say out loud. "Is she going to die?"

"Well, we don't know for sure. We hope not. But right now, we just don't know. We're very lucky, because Mom has very good doctors, and there are very strong medicines that will fight the cancer. But Mom's type of cancer is very serious. Some people die from cancer; some do not."

Lucy teared up and climbed into my lap. I could see the initial shock and insecurity sinking in.

Throughout this process, I think I've tried to make things right emotionally by showing physical support to my kids. I literally tried to make my limbs and torso bigger and stronger when they crawled up on me. While having these tough conversations, I would hold them as close as possible, often with all three fiercely trying to fit under my extended arms and shoulders.

My goal was to ensure that they felt physically safe, even when I couldn't provide the emotional security they were so desperately craving.

That afternoon, I enveloped Lucy in my arms. I think she would have climbed into my body if it were possible.

Although it was a difficult conversation, they seemed to accept our explanation.

I remember thinking that my sadness and worry was palatable. I felt as if I carried the burdens of the world. I felt heavy, as if walking through thick soup.

Cancer robs you of so much. One huge thing it stole from me was humor. We had always had a happy home. We laughed, we danced, we picked at each other.

I have pictures of my teenage daughter with my boxers on her head! The girls and I would play "Can I Come in Your Kitchen?" each night as I washed the dishes. They would line up in the rooms bordering the kitchen and ask me if they could come in. Of course, I would say, "No! You cannot come in my kitchen!" in a loud, Soup Nazi voice. As they ran through, I would chase them with a wet sponge or paper towels. We'd spray each other with water from the sink or hold one victim on the floor for a good stomach blowing session. Lisa would roll her eyes and act as if she was annoyed. But she enjoyed every minute of our buffoonery.

Several weeks after the diagnosis, I said to a friend, "I don't know when the joy will return to our house."

Certainly our children could feel that. They saw me tear up constantly. They noticed that I didn't smile. They could feel Lisa's preoccupation with her illness. For God's sake, their mother who was their lifeline at and after school had virtually disappeared within a matter of days. Their life was turned upside down.

Journal Entry 10-7-09

Tonight I talked to Lucy about Lisa. I told her there would be surgery in December. Lucy thought she'd be well by then. I explained that she would have treatment until June and then more surgery. She cried and cried. She said, "I thought Mommy would be well by Christmas!"

Annie T.'s teacher says she seems to be having a difficult time focusing at school. When I asked Annie about it, she said it's because of Mom. I said why? She said it's a little voice. I said what does it say? She said "well, not a voice but something that makes me think about Mom."

I can relate. I will sit in a meeting and be looking at my boss while he's talking and think to myself, "I can't believe Lisa has stage 4 cancer." It is hard to focus! I pray a lot as do others. If prayer works, we should be set.

I can't count the number of times I held Lucy in her bed over the course of this illness — both of us sobbing. Her petite body nestled in my arms; the dampness of her tears on my chest. My own drippings on her hair.

It's in these tender moments that I came to feel this ordeal had more deeply connected me with my children, more deeply than I could have ever imagined. My relationship with Lisa was stronger than it had ever been before, and I reached a depth of emotion that I did not know I had; one that I'd rather not reach again.

Chapter 16

October, 2009

In October, after Lisa got hooked up to her fanny pack of 5FU, we had weekend plans to attend the wedding of Anna Lee, our former babysitter. Anna was about five feet tall and had more zest for life than most people twice her size. Lisa and Anna were very close. Anna was just starting out, a college student when they met, while Lisa was seasoned with style and grace. They spent many an afternoon discussing Anna's boyfriend, Wade, and if and when he would pull the trigger on marriage. Their conversations were typical Lisa: if there was scoop to be had, she was interested. Anna and Wade's relationship was especially enthralling to her. Sometimes I'd get home from work at six and Anna, who should have left our house at 4:30, was still there trying to keep up with Lisa, although it seemed to me that neither one was short for words or opinions.

I too enjoyed Anna, but babysitters were Lisa's job. The closest I got to really getting to know her was when she had a project for her clothing design class at Meredith College, which was three blocks from our house. She sent me an email and said that each class member had to interview a man who had a distinct clothing style. She intimated that she was impressed with my southern fashion flare, most particularly my affinity for bow ties. Lisa's grandfather died the year before we were married, and her mother gave me three bow ties from his closet. The first time I wore one I received so much attention that I began purchasing more. Within three years, I'd given all of my neck ties to my father and had fully committed to the bow. Anna admired this bold move. Her boyfriend was a typical college T-shirt and shorts sort of dude at the time.

Anna loved our girls and had become particularly attached to Annie T. after spending five afternoons per week with her for a year. Because of their attachment, Anna invited Annie T. to be a flower girl in the wedding. To be fair, she asked Bailey and Lucy to pass out programs. Lisa was tired from her radiation treatments, and I was just plain tired. But that Friday afternoon, we met at the house to ready the crew for the 45-minute drive to Burlington, North Carolina, for the rehearsal dinner.

Lisa spent a few days prior to the big event trying to figure out which dress she could wear that was attractive and yet could work with an IV bag of chemo. She chose a black linen number with a short sleeve crop jacket. She had really cool black and white heels that made her look like a million bucks.

Watching her finagle the IV chord with bra, slip, dress and jacket was quite interesting. She somehow turned the IV tube, which was connected to the port in her chest, so that it could run up toward her shoulder, under her bra strap and out through the arm hole. The entire bag of chemo had to fit through the opening since she could not be unhooked from the drip to get dressed. The jacket covered the lines that draped into a small black cloth purse. This elegant handbag housed her lip stick, sunglasses, Blackberry and…the chemo bag complete with pump and extra batteries. No fanny pack for a formal occasion, even if it did match her outfit.

We were headed down Interstate 40 in rush hour traffic when, for the first time, the pump began to beep. It was a slow beep, much like a fire alarm that was about to dying battery. Of course, we were running late.

I-40, rush hour traffic, an alarm that is attached to my wife sounding as if she is going to explode, and Lisa is strapped into her clothes like a mental patient in a straight jacket.

"What's going on? Why are you beeping?" I asked as if this was her fault. I don't excel in these types of situations. In fact, I sort of freak out.

I always assume I'll end up performing CPR on a stranger. Too many Red Cross classes at the Y I suppose.

"It's OK. Let me read the code," she replied in a very calm manner.

"We may have to cut that dress off of you."

Lisa smiled.

I don't even own a pocket knife. I should be more like my friend Martin. He keeps everything in his car.

"It's not the battery. I think it might have air in the tube."

My mind went wild—

Air in the tube. Air into her blood stream. Air to her heart. Immediate heart attack or aneurysm.

"Should we turn around? Duke is not far from here." I was poised to make a U-turn on the highway.

"No, I'll call the 800 number."

The beeping continued.

"No one's answering."

"No answer? WE'RE HEADING TO THE EMERGENCY ROOM!"

"No, we're not. There's another number. Just relax, honey. I'm going to be OK."

Finally an answer. Fran will call us back.

I tried to lighten up. "I wonder which shirt she's wearing today? Paris or Rome?"

The phone finally rang. I heard Lisa repeating Fran's words, "There's a kink in the line."

"I wonder how that happened! It's probably hooked on your girdle. Ask her if you can die from air in the line." Lisa thought I was kidding.

"Seriously, ask her."

"Fran, Bruce wants to know if I can die from air in the line. Uh huh. OK. Yes, I'll tell him. Thanks, Fran. Goodbye."

"So can you?"

"She said it would take a lot more air than this to kill me."

Lisa dug through her clothes and found the kink. She straightened it out without incident and reset the pump.

We were 15 minutes late to the rehearsal, but my wife was alive — and at that time, that's all I cared about.

Chapter 17

2000 - 2008

I began to get a taste of what life would really be like in a house full of girls when Bailey hit the sixth grade. She was a confident, smart and beautiful tall blonde. I guess all dads think their girls are beautiful, and I contend that most are in some way. But the truth of the matter is, my girls ARE truly beautiful. Strikingly beautiful.

Bailey began to hit her stride in middle school with a core group of friends that I think were trendsetters at St. Timothy's School. Now, how that would play out when she hit high school was yet to be seen. But for today, she was at the top of the food chain.

Because I was a relatively insecure child, I was amazed by Bailey's ability to manage most any situation without hesitation. I recall in high school avoiding PE class in any way possible during the gymnastics quarter, simply because my skills in that area were incredibly lax. Not an athlete, I was skinny and weak. I played basketball in one league during my childhood and remember two things about it –

1. Blaine Parrish spat on me in practice one day.
2. The one time the fourth graders were allowed to play in a game, I made a significant blunder. Being the youngest on the team, we were basically benched for the season. At one game at Horace Sysk Junior High's gymnasium, which to me felt like UNC's Dean Dome, our team was winning by about 30 points. With

three minutes left in the game, Coach Ancherico put the fourth graders in. I was the point guard. On our first play, the other guard threw the ball in to me. I headed immediately down court toward my teammates who were set for what could have been the play of the year when I heard a whistle. I stopped and the ref was looking at me. "Traveling!" *Traveling?* I had forgotten to dribble the ball. Everyone in the gym got a kick out of the fourth grader who couldn't handle the pressure. Everyone except my teammates. It was disappointing for them; humiliating for me. Maybe Blaine spit on me after that game, I'm not sure which came first.

This significant event in my life was a precursor to PE issues for the rest of my school career. Miss Cherry, our Phys. Ed. teacher, called us all by our last names. She was 106 years old and never married. She had short, man hair and wore gray work pants just like my grandfather. One day in class we were running laps around the outdoor track and my friend, Ann McNeill, began wheezing. She went up to Miss Cherry and said, "Miss Cherry, my asthma is acting up, I need to stop." In her typical deep voice, our teacher rumbled, "McNeill, I wouldn't ask you to do anything I wouldn't do. Keep on running. I'll run with you." And off she went with Ann for the duration of the class period. She did the same thing with pushups and arm rolls. "Get 'em up class. I wouldn't ask you to do anything I wouldn't do."

I remember intentionally not dressing out in my gym uniform one day because we were going to have to climb the rope to the ceiling of the gymnasium in class.

"Ham, why aren't you dressed out?"

"Forgot my uniform."

"Really? Let's go check your locker."

Sure enough, I had "overlooked" my uniform that morning which was right on the upper shelf in plain sight.

"I thought so, Ham. Get your clothes on, we've got a rope to climb."

Not only was I weak, I was horribly afraid of heights. I slowly pulled myself up about a third of the way toward the ceiling and my biceps buckled, my legs hanging on to the braided mass of scratchy fibers. The bloody rope burn stung for six solid days. There was no need to complain though. Miss Cherry would have just scaled to the top like Spiderman and told me, "I wouldn't ask you to do anything I wouldn't do, Ham."

Lisa wasn't athletic, but seemed to maneuver life with more ease and poise than I. Bailey was a carbon copy of her mother.

As Bailey's first school dance approached, I was leery of how she would handle the boys. Would she get asked to the dance? Would anyone get asked to the dance? Would it be one big brouhaha — a glob of people moving together, no one paired up at this age? I just couldn't remember — I'm not sure I went to any middle school parties.

Apparently, somewhere on the playground or at the lunch table, Bailey decided she was going with a boy. And she decided that the likelihood of any of the sixth grade "dorks" asking her was nil. So, she set her sights on Sterling Price, a handsome, well-dressed boy whose father owned an auto repair shop. He was an avid golfer with hair so gelled you couldn't move it with a metal rake.

I say that Bailey asked him. Actually, it went like this:

Bailey asked Cameron, one of her best friends, to ask him on her behalf.

Cameron obliged and cornered him in the hall before first period. He quickly responded, "No!"

Cameron relayed the message to Bailey. She was cool with that and quickly decided to move on. This was not some kind of uber crush. He seemed to simply be the least dorky of the dorks.

Apparently in 7th period, Sterling told Kayla, another good friend of Baileys, that he should have said yes.

After school, Kayla relayed the 7th period conversation to Bailey and asked if she should re-ask him on Bailey's behalf the next day. Bailey gave her blessing, and the plan was set for the next morning.

Kayla actually caught Sterling before he left for home that afternoon. He said he'd give her a response the next morning.

In Mr. Wilson's second period class, two other strategists cornered Sterling. "Are you going with her?" Caroline and Dakota pressed.

"Yes! I'll go."

Third period was journalism, and Lisa was the teacher. It was a class of all girls, including Dakota, held in the computer lab. Mr. Wilson walked in and headed straight for Lisa's desk.

"I understand Bailey is going to the dance with Sterling!"

"Oh," Lisa replied unfazed.

Bailey overheard the conversation. "That's news to me! Dakota?"

"Oh, yeah, he said yes! I forgot to tell you."

When they got home that day, Lisa shared the news with me, and it was quite the topic of conversation at the dinner table. I asked, "What does going with him to the dance mean? Are you going to dinner? Do I need to pick him up?"

"NO! We aren't going TOGETHER to the dance, Dad! I'll just see him there."

"Well, Mom said you were going with Sterling to the dance. I don't think that was an unreasonable question. Will you dance with him?"

"I'm not sure."

Had I missed something here? Lisa fully understood what had happened, but I was lost. Is this how the next 20 years were going to be?

I would worry.

They would make a plan.

I would get brought in on the tail end and would not understand what had happened, even when spelled out for me in plain English.

Apparently so.

Bailey was a timid child when she was in her early elementary school years. She clung to Lisa for months at morning drop-off in kindergarten.

But somewhere along the way, she found her legs.

Lucy too was growing into a confident young woman. She is a much more methodical kid than either of our other children. Her room is neat as a pin. She's very conscientious about her studies, and is extremely thoughtful of others, especially her parents.

She is not a pushover. She will convincingly ask for the keys to the car when we're at the mall. "I'll go unlock the car for you, Daddy." When the rest of the family arrives, she has snaked the front seat from her slower big sister and the verbal assault begins. Ignoring her sister's displeasure, she simply responds, "You should have asked Dad for the keys."

However, when Lucy was young, she was much slower to pick up on things than Bailey had been at the same age. I guess it was the second child syndrome. I'm sure we spent hours and hours reading to Bailey when she was a baby. She watched Baby Einstein, and there were few times that an adult wasn't holding her. With Lucy, our time was divided. Now we just had more to do.

One thing she struggled with early on was learning her colors. We worked so diligently to help her figure out this seemingly simple concept.

We would point to something and tell her the color. When we asked her a second later what color the item was, she would not know. I was convinced that our child was slow. Clearly she should know her colors by the age of three.

One of the families who attended Capon Springs with us in the summer had a daughter almost the exact same age as Lucy, and Kylie was a smart, smart child. Frankly, I wanted Lucy to show well at our annual retreat to West Virginia. Showing well for me meant that she could respond to us — sort of like a well-trained dog. If I said sit, I wanted her to sit. If I asked her what color something was, I wanted a similar reaction.

We knew Kylie would know her colors and probably the alphabet too. Lucy had some catching up to do. So in June, we went to work. I gathered 10 green items, 10 blue items, 10 yellow items and 10 red items and put them in piles according to their color. I would point to the green pile and say "These are all green. Green jeep. Green truck. Green block. Green ball." I'd then go through all of the red items. Returning to the green block I'd say, "What color is this block?" "Red," Lucy would say with confidence.

"No, Lucy, it's green! All of these items are green! Green jeep. Green truck. Green block. Green ball. Now what color is this block?"

"Red!"

"Lisa. Something's wrong. She is clearly color blind. Kylie is going to kick her butt on colors."

At one point I discovered that she was answering most of the color questions by saying, "Red." I told everyone in the family, "If Kylie or her parents are around, only ask Lucy the color of something red. She'll get it right every time. But if you ask any other color, she's gonna embarrass us. Stick with red. That's the plan. Don't blow it."

Upon arriving at Capon that year, we quickly realized it did not matter what Lucy knew of the colors. Kylie was off somewhere reading Thoreau while Lucy ate sand and told us that green beans were red.

Lucy was also slow on the uptake with potty training. Bailey learned before she was two. Lucy was still in diapers nearing the age of three, and we had resorted to using candy corn to try to get her to use the pot. One day we went to Ann and David's house for dinner. About an hour after we were there, Bailey, age five at the time, came running into the den. "Lucy used the potty! Lucy used the potty! Can she have some candy corn?"

"Ohhh—Lucy used the potty! Let's go see!" All four adults gathered in the bathroom to see the proof.

Sure enough, there in front of our eyes was a potty full of pee. A lot of pee. Actually, enough pee that it could have belonged to a nearly six-year-old who had drunk a coke and two juice boxes earlier that night. After a short inquiry, we discovered that Bailey struck a deal with Lucy; she'd do the peeing if Lucy would keep her mouth shut and split the candy corn.

I was not happy that she'd lied, but I had to give her props for coming up with such an ingenious plan. I assumed she would grow up to be a fairly shrewd business woman.

As Lucy has grown up, she has proven to be a very bright young woman. She often has straight A's and she is quite adept at keeping up with the world around her. She knows all of her colors and is less likely to pee in her pants than either of her sisters. And, she has always had an interesting and optimistic view of the world.

In fourth grade, Bailey was going on a school trip to the beach. They were going to have some educational opportunities along the way. Apparently one educational opportunity included a squid. After we dropped Bailey off at school, I asked Lucy what she thought they would do on the trip. She said, "She's going inside of a squid" in a matter of fact sort of way.

"What?"

"Yes, she's going inside of a squid."

"Are you certain?"

"Yes. She's going inside of a squid, and Mrs. Peterson (the science teacher) is going with her."

"I had no idea."

On another day, we discovered chewing gum in Annie T.'s hair.

Lisa railed the entire family, "Where did Annie T. get the gum?"

It was a rule not to chew in the house so each of us was a bit scared. I began to think back on the past few days. Had I broken the gum covenant?

"Annie?"

No one immediately fessed up, but after ten minutes of lecture, Lucy finally came clean, "Well I gave it to her but I didn't tell her to put it in her hair."

Apparently that was a decision she made solely on her own.

Perhaps our most intriguing child is Annie T. She has been curious since the day she was born. At about the age of three, she walked in to the bathroom as I was peeing and looked directly at me. She pointed, "Daddy has a tail."

Although I was proud that it could classify as a tail, I felt compelled to help her begin to use the proper name. I said, "Actually Annie T., this is my penis."

She looked at it again and said, "I don't like penis!" and walked away.

Let's keep it that way for a long, long time! I thought to myself.

Another time in the bathroom, Annie T. and Lucy were in the tub together. Bailey and I were sitting beside the tub supervising and talking.

Lucy pointed to her bottom and said, "This is my penis."

Bailey cracked up and said "That's NOT your penis, it's your vagina."

"My bergina?"

I then explained the difference between boys' and girls' parts and appropriate names for all at which time Annie T. stood up with a cup in front of her privates and announced, "I have a big penis!" She's the only one in the family who can make that claim.

Our other two children have always enjoyed entertaining themselves. Annie T., on the other hand, believes being entertained is her birthright.

She has no concern for your sightline to the television if she wants someone to crawl upon. She is indifferent to the computer she displaces as she slides into your lap. And she does not care what else you have going on when she announces, "I'm bored!" with the expectation that you will make moves to reconcile the situation.

When she is left on her own accord, she comes up with some wildly creative stuff. One day she dressed up as Zelia the fortune teller. She proceeded to tell us fortunes like: "Dad, you will take a shower tonight." After a day in the yard, that was a given. She also told me that I would make tacos for dinner and that a cute girl, about 8 years old, would spend the night in my room. But the most impressive fortune of all, in my opinion, was for Lucy. Zelia predicted that Lucy would take her shoes off that night and that she would receive a gift. When Lucy asked what the gift might be, Zelia said, "Your little sister will give you your iTouch back because she borrowed it earlier."

Recently Annie T. asked what paparazzi meant and I explained it as best I could. The next morning she insisted I walk in front of her on our way to the car. I was curious as to why. "To block the paparazzi, dear."

She had created a new persona, half southern belle, half Hollywood starlet.

She's 1/3 Lisa, 1/3 me and 1/3 her Uncle Hayes. A demanding, funny, smart, outspoken kid spun from the cloth of her elders.

Three kids — all special, all beautiful and talented in their own right. Just like any other family, *except* these girls would encounter the horror of cancer in its worst form at a very, very young age. And their scars, like mine, would change them forever.

Chapter 18

October 22, 2009

Journal Entry: October 22, 2009

Week 7 with cancer. At this time life seems to have settled down a bit. Lisa is halfway through her radiation. Her insides are cookin'. She is on the pot for days — she eats — she goes to the bathroom. I think she is losing weight. Concerns me. On Monday, I took Lucy and Annie T. to KidsCan, a cancer support program at Rex Hospital. Helps kids understand cancer. I was in a room with other spouses of cancer patients. Have some weird feelings about this group. It's sort of surreal. Lucy and Annie T. had a great time, so I guess I'll go back. Bailey did not go. She said, "I'm not mental! I'm not going to therapy." The fun and joking seems to be coming back to the house. I'm not sure how long it will stay. I so dread surgery in December— right before Christmas we anticipate. What will they find? More bad news? Another thing we're learning – you can't plan anything. Will she feel bad? When is surgery? Vacation next summer? Who knows how she'll feel from six months of chemo—when will it end?

The silent victims of cancer are the children of those who are diagnosed. Our children were shuffled from pillar to post throughout the fall. I balanced work, the children's calendar and trying to care for Lisa. She focused on her work and beating cancer. Together we went from two very attentive parents to about one half of a parent in total.

A child not only has fears of what could happen to their parent or to them, but they also have a parade of folks picking them up, dropping them off, attending their events with them, cooking for them and tucking them in bed at night. If the cancer alone does not produce anxiety and insecurity, the loss of daily attention and support from your mom and dad has to.

In November, Annie T. went to school with a pair of tennis shoes that had seen their better days. I had not noticed anything about my kids' clothing or appearance in months. While on the playground, a chunk of her tennis shoe fell off. Annie T. took it to her favorite teacher, Mrs. Sanders, who gave her a hug and told her not to worry about it. They laughed and moved on. By the end of the day, Mrs. Sanders had darted out to Target and purchased my child a new pair of tennis shoes. I felt like an underprivileged family and wondered if we would be added to the Angel Tree at the Y — an effort to bring Christmas to families in need.

When Annie T. shared with me about her shoes, she said, "You know, Dad, I have a lot of parents right now."

"Who are all of your parents?"

"My teachers, Nana, Mrs. Janice (her dance teacher), Libby's mom, Mrs. Strickland."

"Do you like that many parents?"

"I do. It's fun. But I miss spending as much time with my mom and dad."

A comment like that can wrench your heart out.

Later that week, Lisa received a good report from the hospital. I think her blood counts were good. When her mother picked Lucy up from school, Ann said to Lucy, "Your mom received a good report from the doctor today!" Lucy said, "Yes!" She then said, "Lunch was AWFUL." It's important that we get our priorities straight here.

Kids have a limited ability to comprehend a situation as serious as the one we were facing. Although a part of me wishes that the girls would have understood how important the next few months would be, another part of me was glad that Lucy's primary concern in life was the shortcomings of the school lunch menu.

Chapter 19

2008

I've read that some marriages suffer from the doldrums about year 14. Ours was no exception. We had always had a strong connection and had so much in common – values, likes, interests, politics, religion. But, the passion and romance had waned to some extent in about year 13.

Lisa and I would talk about it. It bothered us both, but probably more me. She would say, "Honey, this is just where we are in life. We have young kids. They are our focus. We're just at that stage." It wasn't anything serious; we just tolerated marriage mediocrity for a while.

She seemed to want more time for us to relax without chasing kids around the house. I wanted more, well…

She was tired, exhausted from working full time, volunteering in the community and raising three kids. I was tired too and cheap. I worried about finances which put a damper on our ability to hire a sitter and enjoy nights, or better yet, weekends away for much needed adult time.

I don't think I understood how important it was to give Lisa a break, time away from the kids. It seemed that my wife just wanted to eat dinner where we didn't have to bicker with a child over the offerings on the kid's menu; perhaps a meal with a waiter who came to your table versus a cafeteria line where the staff yelled, "Can I help you with your meat, sir?" I don't think she fully understood my need for, well…

We plundered along with life for several years with a window of romance periodically, but more often than not, our primary focus was on strengthening the family, not our marriage. But in the spring of 2008, just by happenstance, all of that changed.

It was in April that I got a call from a staff member at a YMCA in Orlando. He had heard me speak at a conference and offered to pay me to fly down and lead a weekend workshop for their summer staff. I was going to fly in on a Saturday morning and return home that night, and $1,500 richer. I was pumped. When I came home that day from work and announced to Lisa about my new-found bootie, she said, "I want to go with you."

I didn't mind her going on the trip, but if she went and I had to cover all of her costs, I knew I'd spend a great deal of the money I would make, which sort of defeated the purpose of going. In my head I'd already paid off the interest-free credit card bill for the new washer and dryer and knew I'd have some to spare for Christmas. But Lisa persisted. So I booked the tickets.

We flew in on a Thursday, two days before I had to speak. In our hotel room, we found a large coupon book for restaurants and bars at Universal Studios. It was a short walk, so we headed over to eat and began perusing the coupons. What we found were about six two-for-one drink specials.

We didn't use them all, but we did enjoy two or three. We took a cab back to the hotel and when we walked into our room, well, we had a great night! It was an immediate lesson for both of us. An investment in each other led to an unusually romantic weekend and a reconnection we hadn't felt in a while. One weekend and I began to look at my wife in a different sort of way. I realized she was worth my investment. I think she realized that a focus on our family really meant that we had to start with us.

It took effort from both of us, a little communication, a weekend away, and a few two for one drink coupons, and our marriage moved to a whole new level. We were sort of giddy when we returned to Raleigh.

We had always been happy with each other. We'd just let life and work and kids get in the way of *us*. Not anymore.

Our new found passion led me to begin purchasing really expensive underwear for Lisa.

There was a small lingerie boutique in the newly renovated, upscale North Hills shopping center in midtown Raleigh called J. Alanes. I wasn't really comfortable in this setting and had to build up some confidence before taking the bold move to open the door and venture inside. My first visit to the store actually proved to be quite unsettling. I remember when I first walked in, my heart began to beat a little bit faster. I wasn't sure if it was nerves or if I was getting a little excited about the thoughts of what went under their wares. The woman at the counter gave me a few minutes to look around before asking me if I needed any assistance. At the time, she was the only one in the place.

I remember one bra that was pink and had enough room for an enormous set of boobs. There was lace as far as the eye could see and thongs for days. It was high class though. No dangly things from the cups. I had no idea where to start.

The saleswoman came over and asked if I'd ever been in before. I thought, *You have to ask?* My heart still racing and my palms sweaty.

"Nah. This is my first visit."

"What are you looking for?"

"Something for my wife for Christmas."

"What do you have in mind?"

"I'm not sure. A nice bra and panties perhaps."

Is it manly to say panties? That's girlie. What else could I have said? Underpants? Underwear? No, that's what my mom wears. Drawers? Too hillbilly. I'd like to buy her some undergarments. This is not the 18th century. It's panties man, sound like you know what you're doing.

"Well, this is a nice set. Does she have anything taupe?"

"I think most of hers are cotton."

"Taupe is a color that goes with a variety of outfits."

"Of course. She wears taupe clothes all the time. Taupe is actually one of her favorite colors! I think something in the taupe family would be perfect."

It's a color you dumb mug. Taupe is a color!

"Does she prefer a thong or something with a little more coverage?"

"I'm not sure, what do you like?" *Ahh – now she thinks I'm asking about her underwear habits…* "I mean, that's none of my business, I don't care what you prefer. Wouldn't that little string be uncomfortable in there?"

"Some women prefer it. And what is her size?"

"About your size in the bottom, her chest is larger."

I did not just say that.

"Perhaps I have her in my system, let me check my card box."

"Nah, she only wears grandma sort of underwear from Target."

"What is her name?"

"Lisa Ham"

She filed through a box of index cards.

"She wears a 34 C and medium underwear."

I knew I should have said underwear.

"I wear a 34 too." *That's pants man, pants. Why does she have my wife's sizes in her bra card catalogue? Lisa doesn't have any underwear that look like this – do women just go to these stores and give them their sizes in the event some man will drop by and decide to purchase them a thong? What's going on here?*

"Looks like she purchased a strapless bra here last year."

I remember; it was for a wedding. Whew! .

"I sort of like that one." I pointed to the pink one that could hold Dolly Parton.

"That only comes in larger sizes." I could tell she thought I was a pervert.

She walked me over to the taupe line. It was nice.

"I'll take these," I confidently decided.

She thumbed through the small rack and found Lisa's size. She then walked me toward the counter.

"That'll be $130."

What?? It's some lace and 1/32nd of a yard of material. "Great!"

"Put that on your VISA?"

"Yes."

"Hum. The computer is not working. Let me try again."

Several women entered the store.

"It still won't work. I don't know what's wrong, let me call."

Two more women entered the store.

I'm the only guy here. They're all picking out their bras and panties. You really need to hurry.

Ten minutes passed.

"Mr. Ham, if you don't mind, I'll just write down your number and charge you when our system is up and running again."

"That'll be fine."

"Do you want these gift wrapped?"

I WANT MY BRA AND PANTIES AND I WANT TO GET THE HELL OUT OF YOUR BRASSIERE BARN!! "That would be super. Thank you."

My experience at J. Alanes was uncomfortable. My experience there was embarrassing. And, my visit to this weird women's lingerie lounge was the beginning of the most exciting and passionate year of my marriage.

Chapter 20

December, 2009

Journal Entry: December 3, 2009

Today was our first CAT scan since early September. And it was good news! Ovarian tumor appears to be gone—colon tumor has shrunk, we just don't know how much. And best of all, still no sign of cancer in lungs, liver or bones.

Lisa was very tired and sick in early November. She received IV bags of fluid at her treatment one day and was in the bathroom without ceasing! However, she felt great for Thanksgiving and Disney is less than a week away. Surgery is to immediately follow vacation. I promised God I would give him credit when things went well so thumbs up to Him today.

We've actually been laughing a lot lately, which is good, very good!

Every year, St. Timothy's School has a Christmas Pageant. It's a tradition that has been around for 40 years.

As an administrative staff member at the school, and as one who really liked them to put their best foot forward, Lisa took it upon herself to help coach the fifth grade scripture readers for this important event. From what I could tell, the children didn't do much school work from mid November through mid December because they were primarily practicing for the pageant! Lisa expected the readers to project and clearly recite their lines. She was one who loved tradition, and this pageant was right up her alley.

So when Lucy got one of only four female solos, her mother, who clearly gave her the music gene, was delighted. Although Lisa had missed a great deal of work throughout the fall, she kept an eye on the play, and she worked with Lucy at home to insure that she would be comfortable with the song.

The Christmas pageant always made me cry, and I hated that. No other man was in the sanctuary with tears rolling down his face. As the kids entered the small traditional sanctuary, wearing their red robes and processing to "O Come All Ye Faithful," I would swallow hard to hold it together.

Because Lisa had surgery scheduled to remove her gigantic tumor the week of the pageant, the powers that be put on an additional dress rehearsal specifically so she could hear Lucy perform the role of Mary. We sat on the front row; Lisa's mom and dad joined us. Lucy sang clearly, her voice angelic. With brown hair and a broad smile, she was the spitting image of her mother when she was nine years old.

When it was over, Ann met Lisa as she was walking out of St. Timothy's for what she did not know would be the last time; she was in tears. "I can tell they all think I'm going to die."

"You're NOT going to die, Lisa," her mom reassured her.

Her mom was wrong.

Chapter 21

December 8, 2009

Our family *loves* Disney World. I don't mean we enjoy going there on occasion. I mean Lisa and I have collectively been to visit the Mouse more than 20 times in our lives.

Lisa absolutely loved planning a vacation, but a Disney vacation motivated her more than any other trip we went on. She'd start with the AAA books, methodically reading every chapter. She'd then move to the Disney Tour Guide books she'd purchased from Barnes and Nobles. And finally, she'd get online — entering the world of insane women who spent days on end in chat rooms discussing strategies for eking out everything they could get while in the happiest place on earth.

These chat rooms covered where to eat, crowd levels, times of the day you should ride each ride for the least wait in line, and hidden Mickeys. Yes, there are images of Mickey Mouse all over Disney World, painted in the Lion's Den in the Animal Kingdom and hidden in clouds and flowers in the Splash Mountain ride. My wife could find them all.

She'd prepare a color-coded spreadsheet — one that had the park hours, crowd levels and our restaurant reservation confirmation numbers. There was nothing we would miss.

One year, there was a parade at 3 pm in the Magic Kingdom. At 12:30, Lisa said, "I'm going to save us seats on the balcony of the Train Station so that the kids will have the best view of the parade."

"But honey, the parade isn't until 3."

"That's why I'm going now."

"You're going to miss two and a half hours of park time sitting and waiting for a parade? "

"It'll be worth it."

"Suit yourself."

And off she went.

When we arrived at 2:30 after riding Pirates of the Caribbean and four other Adventure Land attractions, there she was, saving seats for 10 – rain coats spread out like bulletins in a pew at a funeral. And the view was spectacular.

Lisa took a quick bathroom break after she basked in our approval.

Two minutes later she returned. She came up to me like a James Bond movie character. "Tell your parents to save our seats. Get the girls and follow me."

"But the parade starts in 15 minutes."

"Follow me," she demanded.

In life I might not have been so compliant, but at Disney, if she told me to move, I moved! She was the expert and knew what she was doing.

When we got to the bottom of the Train Depot steps I said, "What's going on?"

"I've found Snow White, and she's all alone."

Ah, the secret is revealed. And sure enough, in a store right off Main Street stood Snow White ready to spend some quality time with the Ham family.

She greeted us with her big blue eyes, her lips as fat and red as a juicy apple. She hugged each child and asked me, "Who's your favorite dwarf?"

"Grumpy," I replied, not intentionally meaning to offend her.

"That's horrible," she shrilled in her squeaky little voice. Looking at Bailey she said, "I know how to take care of that!" And she planted a huge lipstick kiss on Bailey's forehead.

"I still like Grumpy, but we appreciate your time, Miss White."

"It was a pleasure to meet you."

And off we scurried back to our places.

As the parade proceeded down the road, we saw a float with our friend perched on top. However, I wasn't sure it was the same Snow White. As she came closer, Bailey started waving with vigorous motions. "Dad, she's going to see me and remember me!"

"I'm not so sure, baby. I think that apple may have made Snow White a little near-sighted. She may not be able to make you out."

"Dad, her float is coming right beside us."

And as she rounded the corner, the most beautiful thing happened. Snow White looked up at my daughter, put her finger on her forehead, winked and blew her another kiss.

"I told you she'd see me, Daddy."

A tear ran down my face. "This," I told Lisa, "was worth the $9,000 we've spent this week." And all because of my wife's good planning.

In early August of 2009, my father called and said, "Disney is running a special in early December. There's a great deal on hotels and the meals are included for free. You guys want to go? I think your brother is in."

It was hard for us to turn down a Disney trip, and we hadn't been since February, so we quickly got on board. Although we had not booked it, we had all agreed to a five-day trip the week after Thanksgiving.

When Lisa got sick four weeks later, we debated whether we should go. We had no idea what she would feel like after her radiation treatments. We continued to talk about it and eventually decided we would do everything possible to make it happen. We knew that Lisa would have surgery in mid-December and felt that this would be the only real family time we'd have until after she recovered and completed her intense chemo regimen a few months later.

Because Lisa had cancelled her high school girlfriends' weekend trip to Colorado earlier in the fall, she had a voucher for American Airlines. The girls and I flew down on a separate flight several hours later on US Air simply due to price. This portion of the trip was an omen of my future life. Me with the three girls — Lisa there in spirit.

Journal Entry, December 8, 2009
Picture: Charlotte Airport

Bruce, Bailey, Lucy and Annie T.
Bailey: "Dad, can I have an iced Frappuccino? It's only $4.97. Please, please."
Bruce: "Lucy, stop running the wrong way down the people movers! You're going to hurt someone!"
Annie T.: "I want that pocketbook. Aunt Susan gave me money for Disney World, I want that pocket book."
Bruce: "Aunt Susan gave that money to you for DISNEY WORLD."
Annie T.: "We're going to Disney World, and I really, really want that pocket book."
Bruce: "We are NOT spending your Disney money at the Charlotte Airport during a layover on the WAY to Disney World. No!"

Lisa was bored to death in a hotel room in Orlando waiting for us to arrive. I was about to blow a gasket in Charlotte.

My parents, brother and his family drove down and met us at the hotel. Although it is often a challenge to travel with extended family, with the exception of the airport fiasco, the trip was exactly what we needed. Our hope was to relax and distract. We did not think about cancer one time while we were there. Our minds were clear, Lisa leading the pack. It was wonderful, just like vacations of years past.

When we returned to town, Lisa and I immediately drove to Duke for her pre-op work. We met with our surgeon, and the contrast from It's A Small World to the Duke surgery wing was stark. Lisa had to meet with the nurse who was teaching her how to deal with her impending temporary ileostomy bag. This was their first discussion about what was to come and at the time was the biggest issue Lisa seemed to be facing. She cried and cried about that intestinal bag, a rare occurrence for my wife. I would have been stressed about needles and stitches. She was concerned about the protrusion dangling from her stomach. Lisa was not one to discuss bodily functions, and this was about to put her over the top.

I was typically the emotional one in the family. I cried at the school Christmas pageant and at times in church just because a particular hymn hit me in a certain way. But for some reason, when Lisa cried, I usually held it together. Somehow my system seemed to instinctively know when to man up. If she was going to be weak at this moment, I had to show strength. The least I could do was hold myself together.

The 48 hours before surgery were very tough for Lisa. She was concerned about Christmas, wanting the kids to feel like things were normal. She wanted us to be okay. She did not want to ruin the holiday. As usual, she had taken care of most of the details before she went to Duke, and Christmas morning went off without a hitch.

Chapter 22

December 16, 2009

The day of surgery started early.

Lisa Update, December 16, 2009 9:55 PM
To: Friends and Family
From: Bruce

Hello Good Friends—

Obviously Lisa won't be sending updates for the next few days, so I thought I would bring you up to speed on where we stand. We really appreciate your thoughts and prayers. The support has really been uplifting.

As usual, my wife charged forward with strength and courage this morning and a positive get-it-knocked out attitude. She went into surgery at about 9 am and was in recovery by 3:30. It is 9 pm and we are just getting settled in our permanent room. It was a long, long day for her, but she fared well. She is extremely tired.

She had a full hysterectomy and they removed the tumor in her colon. The surgeons would not speculate about spread to the lymph nodes or about the final call on the ovary but they did tell us that they did not see any indication of cancer in any of her other organs. We will receive pathology reports in about a week.

We did determine that both the ovary and colon responded well to the radiation.

We appreciate your prayers and support more than we can express.

Bruce

Journal Entry Friday, December 18, 2009

Wednesday was a long day. Lisa and I arrived at 6:45 am and they took her straight back. At 7:45 I went back to see her—it took them a while to get the IV in—we saw two surgeons and the anesthesiologist and then they kicked me out. I waited in the lobby alone for a while—which was OK—and then Ed McLeod, Susan Vebber, Diane Hillsgrove, Brad Davis, Eric Caldwell, Ann and my parents showed up. We put our chairs in a circle and enjoyed the time. Lisa's mom and I met with Dr. Lee, the OB surgeon after about 2 and a half hours. She said all went well but that the ovary looked abnormal—

Back up...

September/October: All doctors are 99.9% certain there is cancer in her ovary. Thick mass, "clearly cancer."

12/3: Radiation shrinks ovarian tumor to where it can't be seen on the scan. Dr. Willet and Dr. Uronis say it was still malignant.

12/4: Dr. Lee says "I was never sure that mass was malignant."

Suddenly we have hope that it never was—they never biopsied the ovary because it would not have changed the treatment and because they were sure it was cancer.

PING PONG

Now Dr. Lee says ovary is abnormal which says to me it is malignant. I am crushed. Once again kicked in the stomach although I shouldn't be. I just grab onto this hope, small glimpse—and put my cards on that and when it doesn't come through, I'm back at square one. So I'm so, so sad. Then Sallie arrives and we meet with Dr. Tyler the GI surgeon and he says, three hours after we talk to Dr. Lee, "We don't think the ovary is cancerous." And I say, "Did you say you didn't think the ovary was cancerous because Dr. Lee implied that it was." And then he said, "We just don't know and won't until pathology reports come back next week," and then gave me a long speech about focusing on what we need to do to move forward and not worrying about staging the cancer. He said stage 4 people live and stage 1 people die and blah, blah, blah. I bet if his wife had cancer he'd know the damn stage.

When everyone left on Wednesday at about 4 or 5, I sat with Lisa in recovery. Just the two of us. Long night on Wednesday.

It is often difficult to find things to thank God for in times like these. Lord knows I tried. I thought if I would show my appreciation for the good things I saw, that He would work harder to give me what I wanted — a fully recovered wife. I was thanking Him for anything I could think of, including the gift of texting! Although I was pleased to have this fairly new tool, I'm not sure it was prayer-worthy.

At the beginning of this debacle, at the suggestion of the man who gave me my blank journal, I decided we would keep a list of blessings that we saw during this process. As Lisa and I sat in a small doctor's office waiting for him to arrive, I said, let's list a blessing. Absolute silence.

"I got nothing."

"Me, neither."

"You know, that waiting room was really cold."

"Yep."

"This room is warmer."

"Yep."

"Can that count as a blessing?"

"It's pathetic, but I guess so."

I'm not sure that I will ever see blessings from this nightmare. However, not every bit of it is horrible. There are bits and pieces of good that poke their head out on occasion. Like texting. Or a warm room.

Friends who at Christmas ask our community to send us ornaments for a healing tree. A deeper relationship with my spouse. Now that is one I can fully get behind.

I wanted so desperately to show thankfulness. I also felt that I needed to be strong, that I needed to have grit. It had always been apparent to all who encountered Lisa that she was tough. I, on the other hand, never was.

The challenges I was facing on a daily basis, not to mention the potential challenges that lie ahead, were overwhelming. But it seemed that when she was at her weakest, I was at my best.

Journal Entry: December 18, 2009

OK—stop what you're doing. The ostomy nurse just came, and we switched Lisa's bag. I saw her small intestine—and didn't pass out! Very interesting but not something I'd want to do for a living.

If I never see another small intestine, or large one for that matter, I'll be OK. However, it really wasn't as bad as I had anticipated. When the nurse came in, I took a defensive posture. The nurse removed the bag, and there it was, her intestine. It was pink and looked sort of like the inside of your mouth. Come to think about it, most things I've seen inside the body look pretty similar, just not that shocking.

Lisa Update, December 21, 2009 10:52 PM
To: Friends and Family
From: Bruce

Dear Friends,
Sometimes my wife accuses me of embellishing a story, but this is the truth. I have discovered why healthcare costs are out of control. They have to hire many, many, many people to work the

night shift. Their primary responsibility is to ensure that no pa-
tients or their caregivers sleep. I am convinced there is a monitor
on the patient that alerts the hospital staff of sleep. If the patient
falls asleep, an alarm, a very loud alarm, goes off at the nurse's
desk. She is then required to run to the patient's room and stick
them with a needle. If she doesn't, I believe she gets an electric
shock.

Friday night, between the hours of 11:30 pm and 7:30 am, we
had (and I counted because I could not sleep, no embellishment)
14 visits. There were 12 DIFFERENT staff members who came
through the room that night—some alone, some in groups. If they
average $20 per hour, that is $1,920 plus payroll taxes. Multiply
that by every unit, at every hospital in America—see...

We busted the joint—we escaped. Lisa has had a tough few
days but she was walking and eating and off all IVs by this morn-
ing. They gave us the option to go home today, with a slight bit of
reservation, and we jumped at the chance. I ran to the parking
deck and did a quick drive by. She slumped into the Acura and we
hit the Durham freeway at a fast clip. She's been resting peacefully
for the past four hours.

At this point she is not up for visitors, perhaps after Christ-
mas. She should probably still be in a hospital, but since people
don't really get well there, she will recoup at home. She's in good
hands—mine. I hope her mother does not read this...that might
not be comforting.

We did get the pathology report today. It was confirmed that
the ovary was malignant (an offspring of the colon tumor). She
had cancer in 5 out of 14 lymph nodes—we would have preferred
two but are glad it wasn't six.

Lisa allowed me about 13 seconds to be discouraged that we
did not get an all clear on the ovary and lymph nodes. Then she
told me that if I didn't straighten up I would be kicked off of "Team
Lisa" (our team colors are pink and brown) and she explained to
the doctor the difference between a glass half full person (Lisa)

and a glass half empty person (Bruce). I'm exhausted and have refilled my glass (of wine) twice tonight—does that make me half full?

I can't tell you how much your cards, ornaments for our healing tree, support with our girls (Annie T.'s assistant teacher Mrs. Sanders is playing Polly Pockets with her tomorrow afternoon), love and especially prayer support means to us. I'm not convinced I know how we will get through this, but I do know we have an army out there behind us and that sure does make it easier.

We appreciate you all very, very much.

Bruce

Chapter 23

December 30, 2009

In the middle of cancer, Lucy and Bailey had science projects. It was required at their school for all fourth and seventh graders. How in the heck did I end up with a fourth and seventh grader at the same time my wife was fighting for her life?

This was one of the first real wakeup calls I had regarding my level of responsibility for raising our children if Lisa died. She was the school parent. She kept the calendar, she knew when assignments were due, she wrote the school checks and signed us up for special events. She was the room parent, the cupcake maker and deliverer, the extracurricular coordinator and the homework guru. That included science projects.

I was the tickler.

Sure, I could help with homework if asked. Give me flashcards or a spelling word list, and I was golden. Send home instructions on how to design a science project from scratch, and I was toast.

At one point on vacation a few years earlier, I was dreaming of inventions that could make me rich. One of them was an idea that I still feel could change the dynamics of food storage in revolutionary ways: the Eggspander! Finally, the Science Fair offered an inventions venue, and we would make a prototype.

The idea behind the Eggspander is to save space in the fridge. At its largest, it would hold 16 eggs. As you use two, you push it together into a smaller container eventually to the size of four eggs. Ingenious!

The idea was great. Creating the damn thing was another story. We cut round holes in cardboard. We made it in three pieces that could push together as it shrank. We used a great deal of duct tape. I nearly cut my finger off with an Exacto knife, and when we finished, we had to buy tiny eggs because the Eggspander width was not adequate for the ones we had on hand.

All that, and Bailey didn't even win honorable mention.

Looking back on it, Bailey's project was a breeze compared to my fourth grader's.

Lucy and I decided to test the effectiveness of different kinds of food storage bags/wraps. In order to test, we bought 3 tomatoes, 3 cucumbers and 3 bell peppers. The feeling of being overwhelmed by Lucy's project began the day we purchased the vegetables.

Journal Entry: December 30, 2009

> *Lucy and I went to Food Lion to pick up veggies for her Science Fair Project. On the way to the checkout line, Lisa called. She was taking a shower and nearly blacked out. She lay on the floor in the shower and crawled to the phone in the bedroom. Bailey was home with her, but she did not want Bailey to find her in that condition. I sped home quickly and called the doctor. They readmitted her to Duke. I think primarily due to dehydration. We are on night two in the hospital.*

The stress had begun. Not only did I feel pressure to live up to a science project that would not embarrass my child or me, I was also under the pressure to measure up to meeting my children's expectations for homework support. Lisa not only helped them with their homework, she also monitored their grades. She reviewed their work each Friday, sitting with them to go through each assignment returned to us by their teachers. In elementary school, each child had a weekly sheet that had to be signed by a parent to prove that we had indeed reviewed their weekly folder crammed full of all their work from class. I would look for that sheet as soon as I got home on Fridays and sign it before Lisa had a chance to open their book bags. I'd sneak it back in the folder, right on the top of all their work. She'd get so mad her face would turn red.

"Why did you sign this? You didn't do anything! You didn't even review their work! You just want the teachers to think you're an involved parent. And you aren't!"

In reality, I did not sign the sheet to prove anything to the teachers. I signed the sheet to be a thorn in my wife's butt. Her buttons were so easy to push.

For the science project, we were testing how quickly the vegetables rotted in different types of bags. Because we had to test in different bags and because three different tests were required to prove our hypothesis, we had 27 different veggie specimens.

That Sunday afternoon, as Lisa and I were waiting for the doctor to call and give us directions about returning to the hospital, I helped Lucy prepare for her project. We cut 27 vegetable pieces, made 27 labels for the bags, photographed all 27 pieces individually with their label placed neatly beside, and put them into 27 different baggies. We then put them all on a tray in the refrigerator. It took an hour and a half.

Lisa and I headed to Duke at 5 pm to be readmitted. At 7, Bailey called in a panic, "Dad, Lucy and I walked in the kitchen and Nana had the veggie tray out. She was taking the vegetables out of the bags and making a salad!" I almost swallowed the phone.

"Seriously? Didn't she see the labels?"

"I don't know! She's stressed."

"A science project salad. Did you eat any of it?"

"No! Yuck!"

"Just tell her to put them back in the bags — doesn't matter which one. I'll deal with it when I get home."

I had planned to return to the house late that night to let my mother-in-law go home. Lisa had not spent a night alone at the hospital during surgery, but I thought this was routine and thought she'd be OK by herself. At 11 pm, Lisa had to go to the bathroom to empty her ileostomy bag. It was leaking so we had to change it. Her IV was hurting. She crawled back in bed, and I kissed her and started to leave. She began weeping. It was clear she needed me more than the kids.

Our roles were beginning to reverse. I was becoming the primary parent, and the primary spouse. Up until that time, Lisa was the rock. She provided the comfort for the kids and to a great degree provided direction for me when I was at home. Not only was I taking on a new role in the family, this trip to the hospital was the beginning of the end. I didn't know what was happening, but Lisa was clearly showing signs of decline. Instead of getting better after surgery, she was worse.

My wife had gone from an extremely independent woman, one who managed the lives of three children and a husband, worked full-time and had her hand on every community activity she could find, to physically weak and dependent on me.

Seldom had I seen my wife in a state of weakness. Although she loved me and enjoyed being with me, she never really needed me. That night was different. I'm so very glad I stayed.

Chapter 24

January 2009

I'd talked about a vasectomy for three years. In early 2006, tired of my inaction, Lisa announced that when her prescription for birth control pills ran out in six months, she was not refilling it. She invited me to take full responsibility for birth control which could include vasectomy (her first choice), condoms or abstinence.

Many women talk big about their husband getting a vasectomy. Mine meant business! I tried to pawn it off on her.

"Don't you have some tubes they could tie a knot in or something?"

"Actually, I asked my doctor about that. He said that the next person in our family who should have surgery wasn't me. He strongly suggested you get a vasectomy."

"He can't do that! He's not my doctor."

In six months, I was out of luck. She stopped taking birth control pills, and I was back at the drug store sheepishly purchasing prophylactics. It was a little embarrassing in my early years. At age 40, it was humiliating. It seemed as though I suddenly knew everyone at the local pharmacy.

I resisted surgery but used the time to discuss vasectomies at every social gathering for years. I heard war stories from friends.

One guy told me he still ached from his surgery and that his procedure was six months prior. Another co-worker told me that when the rather large nurse entered the room and pulled up his hospital gown, she grunted loudly. "What did that mean? Why the grunt? Is it the smallest one you've ever seen?"

Prior to 2008, I wasn't sure the positives of this invasive procedure outweighed the negatives of continuing on my current path. However, after our second honeymoon to Florida and our new found passion, my means for holding off pregnancy were really mucking up my style.

The option I'd chosen just wasn't good for the mood.

There were several things weighing on me as I put off going through this procedure. Pain and the embarrassment of the entire medical process were near the top of the list. But my biggest issue was that I wasn't 100% sure I was ready to move from young and able to procreate to what I perceived as old and sterile.

In the spring of 2002, about six months before Annie T. was born, I was on a staff retreat in the beautiful mountains of North Carolina. I'm not sure exactly what the topic was, but at some point in the day, the facilitator told us to go find a spot alone. He then told us to be quiet and to see what happened.

As I sat on a porch, the warm sun beaming down around me, I began a conversation with God. I looked across a large pasture at a mountain. It wasn't big, but it was majestic enough to make you think it was certainly inspired by God.

"Lord, what am I doing? Where do you want me to go? What do you want me to be?"

Silence.

"I'm pretty open."

Still silence.

And before the hour was up, a thought came to me: one day you will have a son. I'm not sure where it came from. It sort of just popped in my head. It was vivid enough that when Annie T. was born, I wondered if we'd have another child — a boy who would fulfill this vision.

As I pondered a vasectomy, I tossed out the belief that that day meant anything. I was essentially throwing in the towel.

Lisa and I discussed a fourth child. Her diabetes precluded us from taking that chance. So in the fall of 2008, I finally made a bold move. I called the urologist.

When I arrived for my consultation, I was escorted by a nurse to the doctor's office. It wasn't an examining room, it was his office with a desk and several chairs. He began to explain the procedure – the thing I most remember from this conversation was his explanation of the procedure, including the use of a soldering tool on your testicles. I could almost smell the burning, like a little boy with a handheld engraving kit.

"Why do you want a vasectomy?" he asked.

"Well, I really don't but my wife won't take the pill anymore. Actually, her gynecologist told her when she asked him about our options, that the next surgery in our family should be mine."

"He said that?"

"Yes."

"Bastard."

"So, is the procedure that bad?" I wanted his full sales pitch.

It did not come. Instead, this middle-aged professional informed me that he would never have this surgery. He said there were risks, that 7% of men had pain for the rest of their lives. He asked me if I could imagine that. I could not.

He then described how he and his wife handled birth control. He freely shared with me that he used the "withdrawal" method.

Did he really just say that? Was this truly a credible form of birth control? A method that someone in the medical field might follow? Was there science to back up this thinking?

I once worked with a guy who used prayer as their family birth control. I suppose that method would call you to pray before becoming intimate with your wife, asking God to allow the sperm to get to the egg if it was His will. Who wants to stop and pray before sex? Who wants to "withdraw"? Talk about killing the mood.

Neither of these is appropriate! Neither should be taught in schools. These are bad options. As God gives us aspirin to ward off headaches, he also gives us birth control to ward off pregnancy.

Needless to say, this was NOT what I needed to hear, not comforting, not in the least. I was more confused than ever.

He asked me pull down my pants. "We need to ensure that you have two testicles."

I assured him I did. But why would Dr. Pullout believe me? He put on his latex gloves and gave me the onceover.

"Well, are they there?"

"Yep. All seems good."

"I told you."

I was thankful a physician confirmed I did have two and that I hadn't been living a lie all of these years.

He gave me a sheet that listed instructions for surgery prep and recovery and told me to make an appointment to be neutered as I left the office. I did not.

When I got to the car, I began thumbing through the information he had given me. The post-surgery instructions said that I would need to ejaculate 10 times before bringing a specimen back to the office. *Let's have a little fun with this,* I thought. I used a black ink pen to change the 1 to a 4 and rushed into the house, proud of my wit.

When Lisa read the instructions, her mouth dropped open. I said, "Apparently the semen has to work its way out and it takes a pretty long time. He said this should be accomplished in about six to eight weeks."

"You have to ejaculate 40 times in six to eight weeks?"

"It's the price you pay…"

For about 30 seconds she believed me, and then my facial expression gave it away. She told me I was on my own for 38 of those.

I waited to set the appointment until January and with a different doctor.

The day of surgery came, and I was petrified. So many things could go wrong.

What if I wanted to have another kid? What if I ached down there for the rest of my life? What if I became excited when the nurse was prepping me for surgery?

It was as if I was attending the funeral of a very good friend. But, I had no other choice. My lack of action was critically affecting my ability to romance my wife. That overrode any other doubts.

Lisa drove me to the office on a cold February morning. Unlike my first visit, we seemed to sit in the waiting room for an inordinate amount of time. Finally, "Mr. Ham." I arose and glanced at Lisa. She was trying to be supportive, but I could tell after having three kids, her sympathy was miniscule.

Nurse walked me downstairs. As we were walking, she said, "I hear you work at the Y! I love the Y. I go there every day. What do you do at the Y?"

My unenthusiastic response, "I oversee several Y's in the area."

"Oh, do you work with the Finley Y?"

"Yes, that's one I work with."

"Maybe I'll see you there."

"Great." *Perhaps you can describe my penis to all of the staff who work for me out there. Shoot me now.*

"Gina at the desk says you used to take care of her kids years ago at the downtown Y."

"Oh. Is she coming down here?"

"No. She stays at the desk."

"Good."

"Now remove your pants and underpants, Mr. Ham."

I could tell at this point that fear number 3 was not going to be a problem. I undressed and lay on the table.

"Just put your legs up in the stirrups."

I'd seen these before but never imagined I'd be hiking my feet up in them.

Nurse pulled out something that looked like a dish cleaner. The one that has a brush on the end and a handle that holds the detergent. She dipped the end in methyalade and proceeded to swab the area like

I would wash my hub caps. She flung it left and scrubbed, then flung it right and scrubbed. She cleaned above and below —very below. I felt minty clean through and through. She then brought out a cloth with a round hole in the middle and set it over my private area where she proceeded to manhandle my testicles so that they would spill over the hole. And there we sat. Me, Nurse and my testicles, red with methyalade.

We continued our small talk for what seemed like a very long time. Finally I said, "Are you going to perform this procedure?"

"No," Nurse replied. "The doctor does that."

"And where is the doctor?"

"Oh, he's probably doing paperwork or something."

I am sitting here scared to death with my boys on display for Nurse to see and he is probably doing paperwork? Couldn't he do paperwork at the end of the day AFTER he has neutered his docket of patients?

Finally, the doctor entered.

"How-How! [The greeting used in the YMCA's father/child Y Indian Guides program]. I know you. You work at the Y. You ran the Y Guides camping weekend last year before you hired Bobby. We just love that program!"

This would have been less painful if I had just attached a fishing hook to my business and cast the line in the ocean.

The procedure was not incredibly painful although the smell of burning flesh nearly brought me to tears.

As the doctor and nurse hovered over me, the thought of the boy that I would never have ran through my head ever so briefly. And then I began to think about unhampered romance with my wife and became convinced that this was indeed the right move.

Chapter 25

Mid January, 2010

Although the start of the new year had been difficult, the surgery seemed to have been a success, and we were moving toward receiving our powerful chemo treatments. Our hope was to begin in early February, the sooner the better.

The only issue we were dealing with was an intense pain that had begun in Lisa's back. It started the first week of January. We all felt that it was related to the number of hours Lisa had spent in the bed. The pain was keeping her from getting up and about and yet, we felt the only way she would improve her back was to get up and about.

I began to put pressure on her to move. She said she couldn't. The more Lisa resisted my push, the more frustrated I became. I really was beginning to wonder if this was real or imagined. She was typically not a whiner, but she was changing. Could this be a sign that she had had enough?

After a week or more of complaining, she finally began to walk some and she decided, on her own accord she clearly told me, to go to a physical therapist who specialized in treating cancer patients. The pain was not letting up, but she was finally making an attempt to get better.

One morning in mid-January, she woke around 5:30 am. I heard her stirring around but was not alarmed. Not until she entered the room and said, "We have to go to the hospital immediately! Blood is pouring into my ileostomy bag." Hayes was there to take the kids. He and I virtually carried her to the car. She was becoming weaker as we drove — she was losing a lot of blood. As I sped down I-40 toward Durham, I wondered if this was it. Could she bleed to death right there on the freeway?

We pulled into the Emergency Room driveway and staff greeted us. They put her in a wheelchair and took my car away.

"Mr. Ham, we need you to complete this paperwork."

PAPERWORK? Seriously? I didn't know my head from my ass, blood was gushing out of my wife's stomach!

"Here's my license, here's my insurance card. She needs help."

Ten minutes passed in the waiting room. A nurse appeared.

"We need to get her temperature and blood pressure."

Lisa was fidgeting and becoming a bit delirious. As they wheeled her out of the holding room she began to vomit profusely. I followed behind. Her head slumped forward.

They laid her on a table and sat me in a corner to watch. Ten people surrounded her bed. I'd seen this on TV. She was still conscious, yet said nothing.

I held my head and prayed.

Pay close attention, this might be it. You could be sitting here with her lifeless body within minutes. Look at her! Pray, pray harder.

I began to explain her condition to the doctors in the room.

And as quickly as it began, they discovered that there was a rip in the part of her intestine that jutted out from her stomach, an easy, easy fix. Two stitches.

"It should never happen again."

"That's it?"

"Yes, Mr. Ham. She's going to be fine. We may need to transfuse her."

"That's it?"

"Yes, that's it."

In a matter of 15 minutes, my wife had gone from bleeding and vomiting, a pale listless body, to chatting and eating vanilla wafers. I thought this might be the end of her life, and now she was eating the snack that they serve at the church nursery?

I was emotionally spent and yet elated that it was nothing.

Her surgeon decided he would admit her to insure that she didn't back track. It had been about a month since surgery, but the back pain continued and got worse.

This short, easy 15-minute fix with an expected one night hospital stay for observation became the nightmare we did not expect as I began to try to dig deeper on Lisa's back pain issues. She had boycotted the hospital bed thinking that it was the culprit of her discomfort. She opted for the recliner in her room. I had to sleep on the beast, and it was not comfortable. Granted, it could move in any direction imaginable to mankind. Feet up, head down? Head down, feet up? Feet and head up? Left arm slightly slanted? Not a problem for this incredible invention. But it felt like you were sleeping on the face of Mount Rushmore with a cheap pair of Walmart sheets. The day after I slept on it for the first time, I felt like I'd had hip replacement.

I asked each staff member who came into the room what they thought Lisa's back pain could be. I was becoming more and more convinced that it was not her lack of movement that was causing this issue. Lisa was not a complainer. She had been poked and prodded in areas of her body that I had never even seen. She had been stuck like a pin cushion and posed on a wooden board for hours on end during radiation. Her complaints were minimal. Her attitude, always positive. But this one she couldn't shake.

As they discussed discharging us on day two after the bleeding, I pulled the intern/doctor/apprentice du jour over to the corner, "We aren't leaving this place until you find out why my wife's back is killing her. I don't know if it is muscular. I don't know if she has cancer growing in there. But we're going to run every test in town until we have an answer."

I had learned that the best-meaning hospital staff could not possibly keep up with our needs on their own. It was essential that Lisa have an advocate. Someone who believed what she told them. Someone who would demand answers. It was a lesson I'd learned too late in this process.

After long discussions and continued prodding, they decided they would scan her back. It would take 24 hours to read the results. I went to work the next morning to catch up on a few meetings while Ann relieved me at the hospital. At about 3 PM I called. Ann answered.

Bruce: "How's Lisa?"

Ann: "She's OK," in a hesitant voice.

Bruce: "Did you get the results of the back scan?"

Ann: "Well, the doctor was here earlier."

Bruce: "Is something wrong?"

Ann: "Lisa, Bruce wants to know if something is wrong. Do you want to talk to him? Let me get Lisa."

Shit. It's cancer.

Lisa: "Honey, just come back over. It's cancer."

It happened again. This was perhaps the worst news of all, and as usual, I was not there with her. Her mother endured the original colonoscopy results. Her mother endured the first conversation about the ovary. Now this.

As I add up my list of regrets, this would be on up there. Although I had put work on the back burner for months, it always seemed to take priority when there was significant news to be shared. Maybe there was a reason things were happening like this. Lisa's mom was strong. Maybe Lisa needed her there to help get through the initial shock. Perhaps giving me time to digest the situation alone for an hour or two gave me the opportunity to play worst case scenario without Lisa in the room. By the time I got to her, I had determined how bad it was and simultaneously figured out a way for the news to be less devastating. Maybe it was just in one vertebra. Perhaps they could remove that one and replace it with a plastic one that could not possibly get cancer. It was still not in the liver. You can live a long life with a healthy liver. That's a very important organ.

I recall returning to the hospital that afternoon. Lisa's mom left quickly.

I climbed in bed with my wife. She was in such pain and the meds were making her drowsy. I held on to her, the emotions poured. We talked about this being the beginning of the end.

"Could this actually be the end?" she asked.

"I guess it could be. But I won't let myself believe that it is."

"I don't think it bothers me that I won't be at the girls' weddings. It's not specifically me that they'll need. It more makes me sad that they won't have a mother, in the general sense, to share their special occasions with."

"The other thing that really makes me sad is Annie. I feel like I have a good idea of how Bailey and Lucy will turn out. But I just can't picture Annie T. in the future, and that makes me really, really sad."

"It makes me sad too."

I held her for just a few minutes. I wanted to put her inside of me – I wanted to fight this damn disease for her. I was strong. I could do it.

But I couldn't. I couldn't do a thing. For the first time in my life, I was not in control, and that was a scary, scary feeling.

The next day I returned home and sat the kids down. I told them the doctors found cancer in Lisa's back. I'm sure they knew it was very bad news. We reviewed the prospect of mom dying.

"I hope she does not die. But she could. And we'll be OK." We listed our family and our closest friends as assurance that they wouldn't be alone.

As I put Annie T. to bed that night, she said, "Dad, I have a question."

"What is it?"

She continued, "Can we give mom's cancer to someone else?"

Her question surprised me.

"Do you have anyone specific in mind?" I was curious.

"No. I was just wondering if we could give it away."

"No, baby. I don't think we can do that. It's not something that we can take out of Mommy. And besides, I don't think anyone else would want it."

She seemed to accept my response and changed the subject.

I appreciated her thinking outside of the box though. At this point no idea was a bad idea. Certainly there was some old person who could use a good dose of colon cancer spread throughout their body. I could readily think of a few.

Chapter 26

Late January, 2010

My wife realized the toll that cancer was beginning to take on me. I was a relatively skinny dude when this illness began — 6' 1" and174 pounds. Since Lisa's diagnosis in September I had lost 20 pounds and was struggling to keep my weight above 155.

The emotional load I was carrying was immense. I was trying to be with Lisa around the clock and wanted to support the girls emotionally as well. I couldn't even wrap my head around my own feelings of sadness and anger, how could I provide the foundation that they needed at that time. On several occasions, I thought I would go over the edge. I wasn't sure what that meant, but I wasn't confident I could go on.

I had always been one who could handle what life threw at me but this seemed to have the potential to break me. The thought of losing control was a burden in and of itself. I could do absolutely nothing to fix this situation. My inability to help my wife, to protect my kids, to save the most important thing I had, made me feel less of a man. I understood that was ridiculous. No one expected me to be able to cure cancer. I realized my limitations. But as a father and husband, there was an internal expectation that I had to protect my family from harm. A job I'd fallen down on.

My beautiful Lisa sent this e-mail to me a month before she died encouraging me to take care of myself. Encouraging me for the work I was doing to keep the wheels on the proverbial bus.

Lisa Update, January 24, 2010 10:41 PM
To: Bruce
From: Lisa

Update: I love you and you are working too hard and you need to go to the State game on Tuesday night. Mom will stay with girls. You get a guy friend and go and then come stay with me. Science fair is almost done and who gives a crap at this point. They can't fail a kid whose mom has cancer. Make the girls sleep in their own beds tonight. Love you L

I guess she was right about the science fair, but I didn't go to the game. I just couldn't be away from her for a frivolous reason. A ball game seemed so unimportant. Deep down I knew my time with Lisa was limited. I didn't quite feel it was imminent that she would die, but I knew in the grand scheme of things, she would not be around very long.

Not only was I struggling to keep the logistical things rolling for everyone in the family and dealing with my pain, I was beginning to have a lot of questions surrounding my faith in God. My father was a moderate Baptist minister. I was raised in a Christian home by two people who were good to their core. They seemed to have a deep, deep connection to God and were supportive in helping me build a strong foundation of faith.

But during this illness, for the first time in my life, I questioned His very being. I felt that the God I loved and worshipped would not have allowed this to happen. He would have intervened and brought healing to Lisa. Literally thousands of people, really good people — strong, strong Christians were praying for her healing. Heck, an atheist buddy of ours had even offered to get on his knees for us. And yet, seemingly, no answer. I could only explain this in one of three ways:

1. God simply does not intervene in earthly matters. He allows things on earth to occur and does what He can to help you cope

and make the best of what you're dealt. He does not, however, pick and choose certain people to heal. Why would He save our next-door neighbor from cancer and not save Lisa? It doesn't make sense.

2. There is no God.
3. The Hawaii Theory

One day I was sharing my anger about God with a dear friend of ours, Catherine Bond. Catherine is a strong woman and someone who I felt I could truly confide in without the fear of judgment. She told me I had a right to be angry; however, she also strongly told me she believed there was a God. She, too, could not explain why He was not stepping in to save her close friend, my wife and the mother of my beautiful children.

After talking with her, I followed up with this e-mail message.

Hawaii, January 26, 2010
To: Catherine Bond
From: Bruce

Catherine,

I feel bad that I shared how mad I am at God right now. I feel really guilty that I'm mad at God. And I'm probably a bit scared He's going to "show me" for my behavior. So I've been doing some thinking about what we talked about today. Here is what I've come up with.

The Hawaii Theory

Say I planned a surprise trip for our family to Hawaii. Two weeks in paradise. The opportunity of a lifetime. I sat down with the family and said, "We're going to Hawaii on February 4!!! Whoa-Whoa! It's going to be great. We're going to have so much fun." And then Bailey, my preteen, says, "I don't want to go to

Hawaii, my school dance is on February 5. I'm not going. This sucks. I won't get to be with my friends, I won't get to wear my new outfit. I'll stay with the Dixons. I'm not going." I, as the dad, say, "Oh, yes, you are! I've paid a lot for this trip. It's Hawaii. You're gonna love it." And I make her go. She goes and, of course, has a great time. Meets a new best friend at the resort and dances with a boy at the hotel teen hangout. Sees and does all sorts of things she never dreamed of. In the end she says, "You were right."

OK—could the dad be God? Hawaii, heaven? The dance, earth? Lisa, the teen? Us, the teens' friends who think her father is the worst because he won't let her go to the dance? The ones who will miss her. The best friend who now has to ride with someone else. The boy who wanted to ask her to dance and had finally built up enough courage.

I'm reaching here. Obviously I'm tired. But...just trying to make some sense of all of this. Perhaps Dad will change the date of the ticket! Perhaps he'll cancel the trip and reschedule in future years. Or maybe, maybe he'll make her go to Hawaii. And maybe I'll have to go to the dance alone.

I know you think I'm crazy. Just grasping for some way to get my mind around all of this.

Bruce

This was one of my kinder days toward God. I gave Him a bye — offering up a theory that made some sense as to why He'd fallen down on His job. At this point and for many months to come, this was as nice as He'd get. I was torqued, and He was the target of my anger.

Chapter 27

January 30, 2010

Lisa Update, 1-30-10
To: Friends and Family
From: Bruce

Dear Friends and Family,

My wife has been a very, very sick woman over the past two weeks. After entering the hospital on MLK Day (1/18/10), we were led through a week of research, testing and discovery by numerous teams of doctors to figure out why a couple of things were happening that seemed to be steering Lisa away from recovery and down a worse path. It was confirmed that there is cancer from the original colorectal tumor in Lisa's spine. We began radiation treatments this past Wednesday (1/27/10) which will help control her back pain. The plan is for her to receive 14 treatments, followed by a CAT scan and a week off. We then proceed to chemo as originally planned. We have learned that a plan is merely that—it can change at any moment. This is a chronic condition, but one that you can live with for a long time if your system responds well to the treatments. I've been told if treatment works Lisa can return to life and work or even travel the world. At this point, all seem like great options.

Since this new discovery in her back, we seem to have a good day followed by a bad one. Yesterday she was awake and her blood counts were moving in the right direction. We even brought the girls over to Duke and had dinner in the family waiting room. Lisa limited pain meds for an extended period of time so she could be "normal" and although uncomfortable, she was a trooper and was caught up on all of the St. Timothy's School gossip and other news.

Today her blood counts have all fallen, and they are testing to see if they can determine the cause. She is tired and resting now. It seems that as soon as we take a few steps forward, something else knocks us back. Yesterday we were talking about a goal of going home on Monday. Today we were told it could be ten more days at Duke.

Our parents and friends have been very supportive and helpful throughout this ordeal. Lisa's closest girlfriends have rallied around her, providing services and a shoulder and just silence at times. Numerous other friends have leant a hand with the kids, with meals and with cards and laughter. My folks are here this weekend making snowmen and leading snowball fights in the yard with the Permar clan. However, what we need the most right now, besides a cure for cancer, is consistency; someone who can take over at home or at the hospital with little coordination. I think we have reinforcements coming by mid-week. Lisa's brother, Hayes, has offered to move in with us for a period of time to help provide this help. He will continue with his sports writing, videos and blogging, which is his passion, but his schedule is very flexible. He can write morning, noon or night. Both Lisa and I are relieved to have this constant coming our way; and the girls all LOVE Uncle Hayes. I'm sure all of you who have been helping us are glad to see another driver and set of hands arrive too! You may see him at St. Timothy's or at dance class, the Y or at church. Just act like he is one of us—

Please continue to keep us in your prayers. We need answers and strength as well as positive response to treatment.
Sincerely,
Bruce and Lisa

There is not a description that can be written that can do justice to Hayes Permar.

Hayes moved in with us in late January 2010, to provide relief during this difficult journey. Although he knew Lisa's cancer was serious, he was living in Washington, DC, and really didn't understand how dire the situation had become. His time with the family at Christmas opened his eyes. He was struggling with finding steady work at the time, so making a move back to Raleigh wasn't as difficult for him, and it was a tremendous help for us.

Hayes' personality is bigger than life. In high school he made straight A's, was a star on the cross country team, played basketball in three leagues, danced and sang in the school show choir, and was President of the Senior Class. He is incredibly intelligent. He made over 1500 on the SAT, at the time I believe acing the test was 1600. He was a finalist for the Morehead scholarship at the University of North Carolina but did not get it. That pushed him to attend Davidson, a stellar institution near Charlotte, North Carolina, where Sallie had graduated a few years earlier.

Hayes was at Davidson for two months when he had had enough. He dropped out and spent the next few years moving from university to university and from job to job.

He is brilliant. A sports fanatic. His mind can hold more information, both important and trivial, than Einstein. He has 1,500 friends on Facebook and dresses like a broke college kid most of the time. He stays up to date on political issues and can argue any given topic like a well-paid defense attorney.

In ways he was the most confident, together individual in the world. From a career perspective, he was still searching at the time. This lack of a 9 to 5 office job was actually a blessing for our family. Hayes was blogging and writing columns for sports publications. This work could be done in D.C. where he lived, or it could be done in a bedroom on Dellwood Drive in Raleigh, North Carolina. Fortunately for us, he cared enough to make significant changes in his life to support us.

Each year, St. Timothy's had a Blue and White Day. When you arrived at the school in first grade, you were designated Blue or White. Once designated, you and every younger sibling who followed you were assigned that color. We were a blue family.

On Blue and White Day, children of all grades compete for points through all sort of active games and athletics. It is the field day of years past.

Since my three children were devoid of the athletic gene, we have not added a great deal to Blue. My kids tended to participate in hula hooping or Koosh ball in the can. Hams leave the tougher sports to others.

Each Blue and White Day, Lisa made it a point to go out and cheer our kids on. It was actually part of her job as Director of Development at the school to attend functions, and she was always looking for a way to connect to the parents. She loved people but also knew that goodwill produced greater results in the annual fundraising drive.

The night before Blue and White, Lucy broke down in tears. "I don't want to go to Blue and White Day!"

"Why, Lucy?"

"I just don't want to go! I hate it!"

"Why do you hate it?"

"I'm not good at anything, and the Blue team hasn't won since I started at St. Timothy's!"

"Lucy, you'll do fine at Blue and White Day."

With tears rolling down her cheeks, "No, I won't. And besides, Mommy won't be here this year to cheer me on."

"Sweetie, I know it's hard not to have Mom there. But there are a lot of kids who don't have parents at Blue and White Day. In fact, most kids don't have a parent there. And Lucy, I know this isn't your favorite thing, but for some kids, Blue and White Day is their time to shine.

Every time there is an awards chapel, who gets recognized for having straight A's?"

"Me."

"And who won the poster contest this year?"

"Me."

"And who was Mary at the Christmas pageant? One of only four solos in the entire fourth grade."

"Me."

"And all of the folks who can't sing, or draw or who don't make great grades have to sit and watch you! Don't you think it's your turn to support the kids who are good at Blue and White Day activities?"

"I guess."

I was kicking butt.

The next morning, I mentioned to Hayes Lucy's lack of enthusiasm for the day's events and her sadness that Lisa couldn't be there to cheer her on this year. He asked me if I was going to go. I told him I couldn't because of a meeting at work.

So, Uncle Hayes proceeded to change his plans for that day. He dressed up in navy from head to toe — blue shirt, blue shorts, blue socks, blue hat and tennis shoes. He even found a blue towel to toss in the air when the Blue team did something worthwhile.

When the time came for the kids to enter the gym, there was Hayes, at the door, giving high fives and yelling his head off. As the games began, he fired up the crowd, waving his towel high above his head, "Blue, Blue, Blue, Blue." At one point he even attempted to kidnap a kid on the white team who was destined to win his heat! The crowd went wild.

The cheering, hooting and hollering went on for the duration of the event, Lucy laughing the entire time, one of only three kids at school with the crazy, cool uncle.

And I'll be damned if the Blue team didn't pull one out for the first time in over five years. I guess the enthusiasm gave them the ummph.

That is Hayes. Smart, funny, the life of the party. A dancer, an athlete, a leader of others. An uncle, a brother. One of my best friends.

Chapter 28

February 6, 2010

By early February, I believe Lisa knew she was about to die. I think she was still open to the possibility of a miracle, but she wasn't banking on that as a significant option. She wrote her closest high school friends, perhaps a warning of what was to come.

Sisterhood Update, February 6, 2010, 7:29 PM
To: Kim, Charlotte, Francie and Susan
From: Lisa

...The final, and perhaps most difficult outcome from January 2010, is how it has left us emotionally, spiritually, mentally. It has showed us that even an already-serious stage 4 cancer could get more so. It showed us that hitting the cancer head on, with energy and good attitude, does not always work. It showed us that looking at things as a glass half-full didn't always mean that the glass wasn't actually half-empty. My role in the family is to keep all of that positive energy flowing and once I was no longer doing that either because I was no longer believing it or no longer physically able to keep it up, we were all dumped upside down. Except maybe my mom, because her strategy works in cases like this—think the worst first and prepare for the worst.

We have for the first time discussed increments of time—what to tell kids, to work or not to work, what's on our bucket list for life, what scares me, what makes me sad, what to pray for, the list goes on and on. I can honestly say I did not think I would die of my original diagnosis, until we found it somewhere else so quickly. I thought there was a good chance that I could go enough years to be considered in remission. And that gave me a lot of positive energy to work through the next 6 months. I don't know what I think now. I think that my benchmarks have gotten narrower, more tightly defined by single days and single outcomes. We will ask work to give me 6-8 more weeks to make some decisions. I will hope to spend more quality time with the kids and Bruce and parents and siblings, improving my physical state should help tremendously with this goal. I hope to taper back on the meds so that sleep, pain and meds aren't the main focuses of my day. What I really, really hope is for everything to go so well over the next month that eventually I'm back to drawing from that original source of positive energy that allows me to Live, rather than Worry.

Lisa

We had been very happy with the care we received at Duke throughout our ordeal. We felt as if the doctors knew what they were doing, and I truly believe that they liked us and wanted Lisa to get better. Our oncologist was young — late thirties. I think she saw herself in Lisa: a working mom, fairly young kids, upper middle class, warm and talkative. I'm sure doctors treat many patients that they have little in common with. Lisa and Hope had a lot of similarities. That made success more important. She did not want Lisa to die.

Lisa outwardly portrayed a very strong persona, but she was not one to stir the pot. If I bought garlic Wheat Thins and I meant to buy regular ones, I'd take the garlics back, even if I'd opened them. Not Lisa. She did not like to make people mad or hurt their feelings. So when Sallie suggested that we seek a second opinion from the hospital at UNC, ten miles down the road in Chapel Hill, Lisa was tentative.

Although this was the place where I had first wooed my wife and her alma mater, she felt an allegiance to her doctors at Duke. I told her there was no reason not to go. Some crazy old friend of Lisa's had suggested a witch doctor in Vietnam, and I was exploring that option. Nothing else seemed to be helping, why not try voodoo?

In fact, a very sweet lady from the YMCA wrote us notes on handmade cards throughout the illness. Lisa loved the fact that Velma wrote about her everyday life. She seldom mentioned cancer in her notes. They were filled with what she was cooking for dinner, the TV shows she watched, what her grandchildren were doing — details of her humdrum life. Her cursive was immaculate. Why did she keep writing us two or three times a month?

We had not seen her since August when we ran into her at the mall about two weeks before we found out Lisa had cancer. As I longed to control my situation and look for solutions, I conjured up the notion (a cockamamie notion) that perhaps Velma was a witch and had put a spell on us. She was sort of haggardly with wrinkly skin and a crooked nose.

If I just get rid of the cards, maybe we'll catch a break. Maybe the spell will be broken.

That thought had crossed my mind on several occasions and finally in early February, as I retrieved the mail, I noticed one of the cursed envelopes with the neat little writing. This had to be it, the only logical reason Lisa had cancer. Yes, Velma had cast the spell on us at Crabtree Valley Mall back in the summer.

I immediately walked to the trash can and threw her note away. Relief rushed over me. I had figured it out. Looking back on it, I realize now the problem was that I threw it in my trash can. It had to be off the property to stop the curse – that, or she wasn't a witch but just a nice old lady who enjoyed writing.

I had gone nuts. I was thinking outlandish thoughts — anything to help put a stop to this wreck I could see ahead of us. For God's sake, I was imagining a dear old lady as a spell caster. Thus, a visit to UNC was a no brainer for me. I didn't care whose feelings we hurt. If there was the potential of someone smarter with more experience, we needed to see him as soon as we possibly could.

Before Lisa could say no to a visit to Chapel Hill, Sallie contacted a friend who quickly got us in to see the GI oncologist. Our young, hip, female physician had been temporarily replaced by a man nearing retirement. He'd been in the business for decades – seemingly had seen it all. All except our case.

After reviewing our files and asking a few questions, he began a conversation that ended like this:

Bruce: "Do you see anything different from what we've been told at Duke?"

Dr. Goldberg: "No. It is *very* unusual for colon cancer to spread to the spine, especially this quickly. I've never seen anything like it."

We are at two of the top GI cancer hospitals in the frickin' nation and neither has seen a case similar to ours??? It's not like we are seeking care for the Zombie Bat Disease contracted only in Somalia; this is colon cancer! The most treatable of all the cancers! And you, old man with decades of experience, have NEVER seen a case like it? NEVER? Good god.

Lisa: "Would you stay the course? Start chemo even with a dangerously low platelet count?"

Dr. Goldberg: "I don't think you have a choice. I would, however, lower the dosage."

Lisa: "And what if the chemo doesn't work?"

Dr. Goldberg: "Then you don't have much time."

Lisa: "What does that mean?"

Dr. Goldberg: "Weeks; maybe months."

Time stopped.

These words coming from a doctor, again, like God Himself sharing your fate with you. I could tell it hit Lisa hard. I knew it knocked the hell out of me.

Lisa thanked him for his honesty, and we walked out of his office together. She looked thinner than ever. She sat in the lobby while I went to get the car. When I drove up, she was nowhere to be found. I called her phone — no answer. Had she passed out? Had she fallen? My mind was spinning. The traffic cops were glaring at me. Finally an answer. She was waiting around the corner.

I helped her get into the back of my Acura TL. She was more comfortable there with her IV bag of meds. It was a quiet ride home. Through glassy eyes, I told her she would not die soon. I told her she had time. I told her the chemo would work.

With all that was going on, I'd never felt closer to another human being. Everyone should experience such closeness and blind dependency. She relied on me for her very existence. I was gladly there to walk her through, savoring every second, fearful that they were limited. I gained as much as she did. Helping her filled my cup as it had never been filled before.

Journal Entry, February 12

> *Went to see Dr. Goldberg at UNC yesterday for a second opinion. I think what he told us was:*
>
> *Your cancer is very, very serious, aggressive and unique*
>
> *There is not a lot of hope for long term*
>
> *You have few options*
>
> *Prepare for the worst*
>
> *Lots of tears yesterday. Held hands with Lisa in bed, cried and talked about the future – sadness and fears.*
>
> *I'm so scared; I'm so very sad. I think I've been in shock since September. Lisa is still on significant pain meds. In some ways maybe that is easier for all of us, perhaps keeps the intensity of emotions down. She says she has the easy part: sleep, some sedation—if she dies she's done with it all. She says that I have the hard part - putting the pieces back together and carrying on. I'm not sure she's right. I guess it really doesn't matter. It's just hard all around. In writing, it seems that hard is not a strong enough word. It is so much more. The prep work for an emotional colo-*

noscopy. I emotionally ache, to the depths, deep, deep depths of my soul. I don't know how much more is in me—is it like snot? You just make more? Or a glass of water that eventually is empty?

Chapter 29

February 13, 2010

Journal Entry: February 13, 2010

Emotional day. Caroline Cheek and Catherine Bond came over. I think there were tears. Lisa wants to go through all of her online usernames and passwords. That put me in a tailspin. We held hands, she rubbed MY back. I will surely miss that.

I do think people are trying to kill me with sweets. At this time we have:

One pound cake

33 chocolate chip cookies

Three heart-shaped cookies

Two doughnuts

Eight cookies in a delivered basket (from my friend Susan; she doesn't cook)

14 brownies

One chocolate pie

Ice cream someone dropped off earlier

Plus two boxes of fudge Girl Scout cookies!

And yet, I've lost 20 pounds.

Journal Entry: February 16, 2010

Yesterday Lisa's platelets dropped to six. They should be above 100. She could bleed to death with a count that low. She would prefer to be home, and doc not pushing to keep her in the hospital. They just say: here are the symptoms of bleeding, if they occur go to ER immediately. I guess if we pushed they would admit her. I emailed the doc yesterday about whether we needed to be admitted for the weekend — I don't think they give platelets on the weekend outpatient. I am fearful she will bleed to death at home—internal bleeding—and I will miss the signs. It's winter break and the kids are going to the beach for two nights with friends. Lisa made sure to individually squeeze the girls goodbye. I think part of her thinks she may not see them again.

Although I know they realize this is very serious, I don't think Lucy or Annie T. have a clue that Lisa is at risk of dying soon due to the low platelets and the aggressive nature of this cancer. Trying to be honest but not have them in constant worry that today could be the last. It could be…or we could have weeks, months, or even years. Based on the tone of the UNC doc, that doesn't seem to be the case but…it could be.

I keep thinking that WE will be the miracle. WE will be on Oprah in five years sharing our incredible survival story. Actually, that won't be the case because Oprah announced this will be the last year of her show. We'll be on Ellen.

Winter break for the children came the week of February 15. Lisa was in a great deal of pain and her platelets had been around 20 on Friday the 12th. She received a platelet transfusion that day, and we were told that it was very unsafe to be walking around in her condition. Most of the time they admitted patients with platelets that low, but Lisa wanted to be at home. She did not want to return to the hospital. After going through this ordeal, I do believe that hospitals can kill you. Lisa must have thought that too.

The doctor warned us that a brain bleed was much more likely with low platelets and to be very careful. Any blow to the head could be very serious. A normal headache could mean something bad was going on.

The inability of the doctors to increase her platelet count led us all to believe that the cancer was spreading and attacking other bodily functions. They would give her a platelet transfusion and her numbers would bump to 50. Two days later they could fall to nearly zero.

I was scared to death. Selfishly, I did not want Lisa to die at home. I felt that would be tough on the children and hard for me. I also felt that having medical staff around would increase the chances of her survival under these sketchy circumstances. If I didn't recognize a symptom, it could be fatal. It was an increasingly stressful responsibility. I could feel the pressure in my shoulders and throughout my body. It was clearly exhaustion in my case: a physical, not just psychological stress. I felt I was nearing the brink of some sort of breakdown.

On Monday morning, all three girls were to leave with friends to head to the beach until Thursday. Three mothers were taking their kids, and they were gracious enough to invite the Ham trio.

I packed them all, and the entourage arrived at our house at 9 am. Lisa got out of bed and wheeled her backpack of pain meds that were being constantly pushed through her port, to the front of the house. All three girls came downstairs.

In true Lisa style, their leaving was not an emotional event. They were going to the beach for four days. That was it. She hugged each one and told them to behave. As Bailey walked up the stairs in T-shirt and panties to finish getting dressed, Lisa watched closely.

"Great, my final memory of Bailey will be her butt!"

"She'll be back Thursday," I assured her.

"I know." She walked back to our bedroom.

Something deep in her knew that this would be the last time she would see her children. This was *the* goodbye. I'm sure she could not fully digest the significance of the moment, but this was it, the final glance at the girls she had carried for nine months and raised for years. The kids she prayed for daily, *God, just let me live long enough to see them grown and happy.* That prayer would go unanswered, and at that moment, she knew. A mother's instinct, I suppose.

The number of milestones we encountered over the six-month period of our battle with this illness was countless. The last Thanksgiving, our final vacation, Christmas, the final embrace, the last conversations — we knew it, we knew it. But we couldn't let ourselves believe it.

She knew more deeply than the rest of us that our time together was limited, and she was at peace. I, on the other hand, was not.

Journal Entry: February 19, 2010

Wednesday Lisa went to get a platelet transfusion and blood work. They told her they were going to admit her on Thursday to begin chemo and to give her platelet transfusions over the weekend which they don't do outpatient. Naturally Lisa told them that was not good and that they needed to fix the system of no transfusions outpatient on the weekend.

What's wrong with medical care? Instead of giving transfusions outpatient over the weekend, they admit you for three days!

The doctor said "We are very nervous about giving you chemo with your platelets this low. This is very risky. We have NEVER given chemo with platelets this low..." NEVER? REALLY? These are words you just don't want to hear from your doctor. "I've never seen..." "I've never done this before..." I was very, very concerned. It seemed like we were going to shoot the chemo in and hold our breath that she wouldn't bleed to death. Here it is two days later and in fact, she may be bleeding to death in her brain right now. How did we get to this point? She's awake, sort of, in a chair beside me. We talk some but mostly not. What is there to say?

She looks tired—raccoon eyes, no color in her skin, dye growing out of her hair, and yet she's still beautiful. I just sit and watch her sleep, it's like a movie to me. At times I can't seem to take my eyes off her. Maybe I fear this is the last time I'll see her.

Bruce: "Honey, is there anything else we need to talk about?"

Lisa: "I'm sure there is but I can't right now."

Bruce: "You're too groggy."

Lisa: "Yes. Do you want me to read that letter you wrote?"

Bruce: "Nah, you couldn't, I scribbled it."

Lisa: "How was I ever going to read it?"

Bruce: "I was going to type it or read it to you. Basically it says you are a good wife and a good mother."

Lisa: "I think I believe that."

Wednesday we had to decide what to tell the kids. They were still at the beach — I called them. Jill, one of our dearest friends, answered the phone. I told her Lisa was going back to Duke. She got emotional and offered to bring the kids back that night. Lisa did not want that. I told Bailey Mom was going back to the hospital, there was a new drug they were giving her that was very strong and they wanted to monitor her. That it could help or hurt.

Talked to Annie T., she asked, "Why is Mom going to the hospital again?"

Me: "They are giving her a new drug — they hope it will help her but it is very strong and they don't know if it will."

Annie T.: "What if it doesn't?"

Me: "We've talked about that. Mom could come back home still very sick, or she could die."

Annie T.: "OK."

New subject.

Talked to Lucy —

Me: "Mom's going back into the hospital tomorrow.

Lucy Powell started crying.

Me: "They are trying a new drug and need to watch her very closely."

LP through tears: "OK."

Lisa called out from the bathroom: "Does she need to talk to me?"

Me: "Do you want to talk to Mom?"

LP: "No."

It was just too hard to hear her voice.

Lisa had been so weak that her voice was soft, very difficult to hear. She had been so drugged up that at times her tongue was thick. It was hard for me — it was very hard for our kids.

Thursday we felt a bit better about our impending date with chemo after talking to Dr. Uronis. She was serious but did not imply a much greater risk than what we were already facing.

Took us four, maybe five hours to check into the hospital.

That night, right before they started the chemo, Lisa said, "I don't know if I'm strong enough for this."

"Should we wait?"

"I just feel like we're doing something big here."

"Baby, we'll get through this." I'm not sure I believed myself.

Journal Entry, February 19, 2010

It's Friday. Today they discovered a small brain bleed. I feel like we may be near the end. She's very tired, achy, still beautiful. I just want to hold her like I used to in our bed. I don't think I will again.

Last night she said she didn't want to live like this—sick, disoriented, unable to be what she used to be.

I feel guilt—tons of guilt—to feel the same way. But this is not good; it hurts too much. I long for my complete family, God give them back! I'll never take them for granted again.

Don't let her die. Don't let her live like this.

Chapter 30

January 19, 2010

I had never been an arguer. I had drive and liked to get things my way, but arguing was never something I enjoyed. I'm not sure that it was healthy, but growing up, I never saw my parents argue. On occasion, when my dad would use a harsh tone with my brother or me, my mom would jump in to save us.

My dad would use words like asinine or idiotic when my brother or I did something he didn't agree with. My mother would follow with "Now, Wayne, I believe this is what Bruce meant when he did that. Your tone is a little harsh." My dad would spout off a few more sentences and then back off. He didn't fuss at us often, and seldom did he use that tone with mom.

My father-in-law is a bit like my dad. However, David is more likely to express his opinion and argue you down on an issue.

"You need to have all of your money at the Credit Union," he'd tell me.

"I have most of it there, but I really like First Citizens."

"That's not the best place for your money. The interest rates at the Credit Union are better."

"I don't have much money at First Citizens, and it's convenient. Plus I have all of my online stuff set up there."

"You need to change it!"

"I've done the math comparing the two banks. If I switch my money, over a lifetime I will make 49 more dollars in interest at the Credit Union. It's not worth it to me. Besides, the banker at the Credit Union wears a black suit with a dark red shirt. I don't like that. It looks like he should be working in a casino. It doesn't give me confidence. If they can't dress appropriately for work, how in the world can they take care of my money?"

"We have different financial strategies! You don't value every penny!"

I didn't even know I really had a financial strategy. I sort of took that as a compliment.

Lisa got her ability to argue from David, and I'm not sure that was a bad thing. A little fussing sort of kept things on the table in our relationship. Left to me, we would have simply smiled at each other and gone to bed at separate times.

Early on in our marriage, when Lisa and I would disagree, and Lisa would get annoyed with me, I assumed we were on our way to divorce. That was not the case. She just liked to dig her heels in. I slowly learned to take up for myself, but it took a lot to get me riled.

This disease, however, yanked my chain. In fact, it shook the hell out of me. There was no human for me to fight with — no one had any control. So I began to take my frustrations out on God. I was cautious at first believing that if I behaved, God would be more prone to meet our needs. I sort of treated Him like Santa Claus. If I was a good boy, a faithful and strong Christian, my original assumption was that He would deliver Lisa from this illness. If he did, I would go on the road and repay Him by promoting His healing abilities. I questioned from the get go, but I didn't start out disrespectful toward God.

As Lisa's health worsened, I began to lose my ability to hold my temper. I specifically told Him I could not pray for His will to be done because I feared His will was to take her from us. I had people tell me that God would work this out. That He was in control. That He may not answer my prayers the way I want him to but that He was there for me. That was of little consolation.

Daily, often multiple times each day, I would kneel on the floor, something I'd never done before, to show my reverence for Him. I would beg from the deepest parts of my being for God to make Lisa physically well. I would cry out in pain. I would make promises. I would fall lower and lower, head bowed, tears flowing, anguish gushing from my heart.

And then, the week before Lisa died, I gave in.

She was so very sick – in so much pain. Her mind was fried with the meds. She was nervous and fidgety. She could not get relief. It was pathetic. She could not move around easily. Going to the bathroom was difficult; a shower next to impossible. This was not living.

Many fathers have a designated chair that they sit in to watch TV. My grandfather's was a large goose neck rocker covered in brown Naugahyde with a small, square matching ottoman. As a kid, when I sat in the chair, my hair would get caught behind the buttons holding the fake leather in place. When I stood up, it would hurt like hell.

After Granddaddy Ham died, I asked for the huge piece of furniture. Lisa was not a fan and could not see the potential that lay beneath the dusty plastic. After years of storage, we brought it out and recovered it in bright orange fabric, my choice. We put it in our bedroom and it looked cool; a unique piece, updated and snazzy.

It was February and by 7 pm it was dark outside. I walked into the bedroom after arriving back home from Duke, Sallie was on Lisa duty. Overflowing with emotion, I knelt down placing my upper body over the pumpkin colored ottoman.

"Goddamn it. You've won!

"Uncle!

"This is no way to live.

"You should be ashamed of Yourself! Look what You've let happen. She is not my wife anymore. You've taken that from me.

"It's clear You aren't going to fix this situation. You are going to let my beautiful wife and the mother of my children die. You are going to leave me here alone. I hate You!

"But if You are not going to heal her, if You *cannot* make her well (a little dig at His lack of power), then take her. YOUR WILL BE DONE! I CANNOT WATCH HER LIKE THIS ANY LONGER!"

I bellowed.

And then I gave Him an ultimatum, "But if You do take her from me, Your ass BETTER walk beside me to get me through."

Yes, I said "ass" to God.

And that was it. I gave in. I prayed the prayer that all of my evangelical friends wanted me to pray. If what they said is true, I guess that night I fully submitted to God's plan. But it wasn't pretty. I did it on my terms, not His.

Chapter 31

February 20, 1010

Journal Entry 2-20-10

> *Yesterday they found a brain bleed. Complaining of a head-ache on Thursday night, pm doc gave Tylenol after I brought the headache to their attention and said "Couldn't this be a sign of a brain bleed?" In the morning the day doc, Dr. D., ordered a CT scan, and they found it.*

Now I'm no physician, which is my point here, but it is crazy that I discovered that my wife had a brain bleed. They kept sending her home, for two whole weeks, with platelets below 20. I was told it was very dangerous to walk around with platelets below 20 and to keep a close eye on Lisa. If she bumped her head in any way, I should rush her to the hospital. In addition, a headache was a sure sign of a brain bleed that could easily kill her.

So, after a day of complaining about her head hurting and sharing it with the nurse, I asked for the doctor to come to the room to discuss her situation. Not only was she continually complaining about her head aching, she was complaining while doped up on a medicine shelf full of pain killers! If your head hurts while on a significant amount of pain killers, something is not right! But what do I know? I just work at the Y.

Journal Entry 2- 20-10 cont'd.

At first it seemed ominous. Then last night the neuro guy acted like it wasn't a big deal, so much so that I went home and left Sallie with Lisa. This morning, it became a huge deal again. They are moving her to Neuro ICU.

Sallie just left. Last night Lisa was alert for a couple of hours. She wrote Bailey and Lucy Powell a short letter and then was out of it. It's noon, and fortunately she woke up and became alert enough to share a few more thoughts about them and have me write some words to Annie T.

She also scripted some ideas, through me, on house rules she wanted the girls to follow when she was gone—particularly focused on getting along and supporting each other.

I then lay in bed with her and read to her a letter I had written. She was tired but listened and told me it was good—to put it in the book with the notes to the girls.

Several weeks before this day, I had written a letter to Lisa in the event she died. I desperately wanted to share it with her to help her understand exactly how much I loved her, how proud I was of her, and to point out all of the accomplishments she had made to our world. I saved it until that day, and it was one of the last meaningful things I said to her.

In order to read the letter to Lisa without interruption, I had to ask the nurse to put a "Do Not Disturb" sign on our door. I climbed in bed and told her how much I loved her. She was so tired and weak.

After reading her the letter, she asked me to take out a pen and a piece of paper. I was anticipating something prophetic to come out of her mouth. Perhaps she would share her deepest feelings about me. Maybe she had advice about raising the girls on my own. She'd certainly tell me what a great husband and father I was.

"Write each of the girls' names down the left side of the sheet of paper. Now, get out the calendar. Write each week of the summer across the top of the paper. I want to go through the girls' summer schedule with you. You can use this as a guide for planning summers for the next few years."

In her state of delirium, near her deathbed, my wife wanted to be sure that I knew what in the heck was going on this summer with our kids. Rightly so, she was concerned that June would appear, and I wouldn't have any idea that we needed childcare.

She rattled off all of the camps and vacations that we had on the calendar. She told me which child's friend was also slated to sign up so that they didn't have to go it alone. She suggested that I call a close friend, Maura, for assistance with carpooling and to help cover the few days we didn't have camps for Annie T.

I dutifully wrote down the information.

Journal Entry 2-20-10 cont'd.

She told me she wanted to give me permission to get remarried—she told me to put in writing for the girls to support me in my decisions but that I needed to talk with them if I "visited"/ dated or even married someone else. I told her I did not want to write that. She said "Then bring the pen to me." So I wrote it.

At certain moments, like last night, I feel I'm getting emotionally stronger.

12:50 pm

My parents just came by to bring my phone charger. Don't know what the future will bring but for them and for Lisa, this was goodbye. Mom sat on her bed, Dad held her hand. Lisa told them that they raised a good boy and that they have been so good to her. Dad talked about Annie T.'s basketball game this morning. Mom cried. I cried. I am amazed at what Lisa can say with no tears. She told them she thought this was near the end. I said not necessarily.

I wonder on which page of this journal that I'll finally write "She died"? In three pages? 30? Will it be in the next journal? Will I die first? Hopefully, in my eighties.

Lisa just reminded me we were engaged on February 20. I asked her if she really looked in my coat pocket for the ring when I went to the bathroom on the night we were engaged. She said yes, but just for the box, says she didn't look at the ring.

Three times during this cancer journey I have thought my wife could die.

When we entered the ER at Duke with the blood pouring into her ostemy bag. I sat in a small chair in the room with her—she was bleeding and vomiting as we entered the ER. Frightening hour.

During our marathon 19-day stay, on about day five, Lisa's heart rate increased to 177 and would not go down. Her arm was on her chest, and I could see it bobbing up and down. Nurses and doctors came running in. It was a scary madhouse. Today. Although she has just been sleepy, not any real signs of stress, but the doctor this morning said this is very serious, "we'll do what we can."

And yet, for now, she seems stable. She's tired and feels like crap but she seems stable.

Our conversation in her bed that morning would be the last normal conversation with my wife. I wish I had done more to maximize the time.

We woke up knowing about the brain bleed, but after the last visit from some young twerp in scrubs, had assumed we had little to fear. Her platelets were up, and we were well on the mend. Boy, were we wrong.

Shortly after awakening, our room was buzzing with staff. Three people from neuro greeted us with horrifying news. The one male in the group began the conversation.

"This brain bleed is very serious. We are moving you to Neuro Intensive Care as soon as we have a room available. We will do all we can."

"But last night we were told this wasn't a big deal."

"Who told you that?"

"Some dark-haired young dude who acted as if she had scraped her knee."

"Mr. Ham, this is very serious. All I can tell you is that we will do all we can."

The physician on the hall came to the room and took down the chemo IV. "We'll hook this back up when we get this bleed under control."

The nurse began an eight-hour infusion cycle of platelets, followed by fluids, followed by blood, followed by platelets. They put more stuff into my wife than came out of me on the night of my colonoscopy prep. Our nurse was literally in our room every 15 minutes for the duration of the day changing out a different infusion bag.

At one point in this long, long day, I began to think about funerals. What would we do for her? How could we honor her?

I couldn't go there because it was admitting defeat. It was succumbing to the disease. I still believed we could win.

Journal Entry: February 20 cont'd.

Funeral or actually Memorial Service? I don't think you have a funeral if you are cremated. I don't think I can clearly talk about Lisa's demise, so I thought I might write about mine. What would I want at my memorial service?

Rather than a hand shake line at a funeral home or in the fellowship hall at the church, what if we opened our house up, served beer and wine and let folks float in? It would be a drop in – like a party but with a crappy theme.

Journal entry, February, 20 cont'd., 4:35 pm

She wanted me to sit by her side a few minutes ago. I held her hand, she is so uncomfortable and agitated (that is the drugs). She told our doctor who dropped by that she wanted to know who to talk to when she was ready to give up. I told her if she was ready to go, that although I did not want her to, I would handle things here — that she could go.

I think I expected that to be it, last breath, movie stuff. She's still here thank goodness. I believe it is the steroids talking.

Journal Entry: February 20 cont'd., 9:20 pm

We've moved to Neuro ICU. This is a crazy place. You walk in and there are rooms with sliding glass doors. All are wide open: patient on bed in the middle, huge contraption from the ceiling to floor behind the bed with all kinds of metal appendages. You can see every very, very sick patient. There is a toilet in the back corner, no curtain or door around it. A TV, a window. All sorts of motors running and beeping. It sounds like a factory.

Ann and David came over tonight—came in to see Lisa, one at a time then we sat in the lobby of the fourth floor talking about life, death, Lisa's Memorial Service, Hospice, where to die. We ate downstairs in the cafeteria and talked some more. In ICU I can't see Lisa from 2-4, 7-8:30 pm, and 11 pm–8:30 am. There is a lobby, not very big or nice, that I can wait or sleep in. It's actually not a lobby; it's a small waiting room. I'm not sure where I'm going to sleep or IF I'm going to sleep. I pondered going home but got a very strong sense from Ann that I needed to be here — she's probably right. But I'm already tired and it's just 10 pm. It will be a long, long night.

I loved our nurse, Seana, today. She was incredible. Competent and yet very caring. I told her she was our angel.

Lisa seemed ready to give up today. I don't think it's time yet. We need to get through this brain bleed but if we do, I don't see any reason why we shouldn't follow through with chemo. She has cancer in her spine we know and a small bit in the chest but it isn't in a lot of places. We don't want to sit waiting for the cancer to spread not doing anything about it! Now if they say — it's spread, we can't help anymore, that's one thing.

Neuro doctor, I repeat, Neuro just came by asking us a bunch of questions about what meds she's taking. We started going through them and finally he walked away and picked up her chart and said, "I'm going to go read." You think??? I'd have thought your ass would have "gone read" an hour or two before we rolled down here! We waited eight hours to get here—couldn't you have "gone read" at some point during the day?

Sometimes I think there are monkeys running this place; except for Dr. D. — he's the exception.

I look at her now, in ICU. It's about 10 pm. At 11, I'm sent out until 8:30 am. Will I see her again alive? 9 ½ hours apart doesn't in many regards seem long. Tonight it will feel like a lifetime. As I read that sentence, it seems like something from a romance novel — "Tonight it will seem like a lifetime." But, in many regards — there could be a lifetime before I see her again. If there is heaven, and I think there is — I guess, perhaps one day we'll be together again.

Is there heaven? If Lisa leaves tonight, what do I believe?

Looking back on it, I am floored at how quickly Lisa's condition worsened between 4:30 pm on the 9th floor and 7:30 pm on the fourth floor. Late that afternoon, we had a conversation, and she stood up and walked to the bathroom alone. I kept a close eye on her, but she independently moved from the bed to the bathroom and back. She also brushed her teeth.

She was wheeled down to ICU at 5, and I was told I had to leave so that they could get her situated. I gave her a kiss, and they rolled her in.

When I returned at 8:30, she could not stand. She had a look of fear in her face. "Bruce, I can't stand!"

"What do you mean you can't stand?"

"My legs, they won't work. They won't support me. I can't control them."

She sat up and tried to stand with me by her side. Her legs were like spaghetti. The nurse brought in a bed pan because she had to pee. She sat on it but couldn't. This activity repeated itself about six times. Finally, they inserted a catheter.

I saw my wife failing before my eyes, so much so that they allowed me to stay in her room the whole night.

I believe she began the process of dying that afternoon. Her body could no longer function. Cancer and its side effects were taking over. There wasn't anything that anyone could do to help.

Chapter 32

February 21 – 23, 2010

Journal Entry: Monday, February 22, 11:50 am

Left the hospital yesterday fully exhausted, physically and emotionally. Got home and rode my bike to the playground at Lacy Elementary School with Lucy and Bailey. Annie T. rode her bike on Dellwood Drive with Pops 'cause she just learned to ride on two wheels.

I think Annie T. is pulling away from me a little bit. I imagine it will be temporary and is due to my absence. She is less happy and cuddly than she used to be. When I got home my plan was grocery store, get the kids to church and then sleep for a long night. But...I got a call from Tony, our ICU nurse, asking if they had permission to intubate Lisa if needed. After a shower and dropping the kids off at the Bonds house, I tried to take a nap just to give me some juice before returning to Duke. I woke up in 15 minutes having what I would consider an anxiety attack. I felt weird—pacing, not knowing or seeing a way out of this situation. Sort of a fear of losing my sanity.

I called my parents and told them I wasn't right. We talked through it and determined that I should not go back to the hospital. I had to sleep and that Mom and Dad should immediately come to Raleigh. I called Sallie, who was with Lisa, and told her I thought I should stay home and rest and she agreed. I felt a little better, took a sleeping pill and slept for 10 hours.

This morning I returned to Duke, and Sallie and I called her parents and Hayes in to discuss the order for intubation, Do Not Resuscitate, etc. I sort of began to have another anxious moment and am now at my doctor's office to get a prescription for some-thing that could help me. We'll see what he says. Am I on the cusp of a breakdown? What is that? What does it look like?

Throughout my life, I had encountered people with mental illness. Supervising hundreds of staff members through the years in my work, hearing stories about nutty third and fourth cousins, offshoots of my 21 great aunts and uncles, made me aware that there were people who struggled with handling life. That, however, was not me. I handled things – and handled things well. I had no anxiety, no lack of control.

I remember waking up from my short nap that Sunday night and pacing around the house. I was walking in circles, and my mind was unclear. I couldn't lie down. I could not put together a coherent thought. My mind was racing, *What am I going to do?* For the first time ever, I had no control of myself or my thoughts.

I remember calling my parents and speaking very slowly. It was all I could do to get the words out of my mouth. I believe at that moment, I briefly considered killing myself. I could not reason another way out. I could not see life without her. I was exhausted and overwhelmed. I felt the weight of the world on my shoulders.

I so wish I could have been stronger. I so wish I would have rushed back to the hospital to be beside Lisa. Why did I leave her? What was so important at home that I couldn't leave the house to help her? How could I leave Sallie with all of that responsibility? Why couldn't I have controlled my mind?

Looking back on it, I believe that was my weakest hour. I do not have a ton of regrets, but this is one. I felt as though I let her down.

Journal Entry: Monday, February 22, 5:30 pm

The doctor gave me a long-term antidepressant with an anxiety component and a fast acting drug, Xanax. I took half of that, and it seemed to calm my nerves a bit. I'm back at the hospital in the room with Lisa where I should be.

Hayes texted me: 3:44 pm

She may surprise us yet. Hang in there man. How's that Zany bar?! (Xanax reference) I could've gotten you those without prescription…I am by no means calling anyone else a doubter, but I think I may still have the most hope she's going to get better. Well, me and Lucy. I think she may.

Sweet, sweet brother who was connected to her like none of us. They really had a very special relationship.

Hayes had hope. He had hope that most of us had lost.

As we began to grapple with making decisions about how to proceed, very difficult questions were coming our way. Did we give the doctors the nod to intubate? I didn't even know exactly what it meant. Did we allow them to put in a feeding tube? Did we want a ventilator? The implications of any could be the deciding factor on how long we had our Lisa.

I'd never had to make life or death decisions. I guess some people do that on a day-to-day basis in their jobs. Not me. The pressure was mounting.

We called a family meeting at the hospital. Lisa's parents, Sallie, Hayes and I gathered to begin to prepare for what might be next. Sallie worked to help us understand the medical issues that we were facing and to clarify the language and repercussions of action or inaction. I listened intently. I had laser beam focus.

Our family worked seamlessly to talk through the situation and to look at options. I believe that Hayes, being my new roommate and co-parent, had the strongest understanding of my fragile state. He worked diligently to help lift my load. I remember he told me he had full confidence in my ability to make the right decisions and that he knew I had his sister's and nieces' best interests at hand.

Not once in the time leading up to Lisa's death did I ever feel a sense of distrust within our family. Her parents were wonderfully supportive — sharing ideas but not overpowering me. My parents took a backseat, helping whenever possible but not wanting to intrude on Lisa or her precious time with me, her family or the girls. Sallie flew in from Boston over and over to give me a respite, and we talked daily about Lisa's condition. And Hayes? He not only took over many of the logistics of our home, he became my confidante and my shoulder to cry on. He became a parent when I just didn't have it in me. And on occasion, as time progressed, he gave me a kick in the butt when I wasn't living up to the father, or the person, I was meant to be.

Chapter 33

February 23, 2010

Journal Entry: Tuesday, February 23, 4:55 am

Lisa has not been awake since I got back in the room at 8:30 pm. John, our nurse, tried to wake her earlier. She wouldn't squeeze his hand but did move her toes. He said her lung scan looked the same. Could this be congestive heart failure?

Sunday she was writing on a pad a bit because she had a huge breathing mask on. She wrote at one point:

I want the option to get out at any time.
L. Ham

I think we all know what that means.

Yesterday as I worked to get her oxygen mask on her while she was aggressively pulling it off, she said:

"You did this to us!"

I don't know if that was crazy talk or a reference to the fact that I was the one who pushed to get her readmitted to the hospital at the end of last week.

But is she better off here?

I was not at the hospital when Lisa began writing in a small journal that her mother left in the room to communicate. She could no longer talk.

Not only did she write that she wanted the option to "get out" at any time along with her simple, cursive, L. Ham signature, but she also wrote at various points that afternoon:

"It's so ugly."

"Bad price!"

"Limited function!"

"Ugly atmosphere!"

Lisa loved word puzzles. She began writing down letters and trying to get Sallie to guess what they stood for.

POC — *Pirates of the Caribbean*

SWAC — *Sonny with a Chance*

ROTLA — *Raiders of the Lost Ark*

And the last one, very appropriate for Lisa:

IASWAA — *It's a small world after all.*

This was the afternoon that I was having my anxiety attack — unable to be there for her last day of interaction because I was dealing with *my* personal meltdown. What a waste.

I have struggled with Lisa's last words to me, "You did this to us." There are so many other things she could have said like: "You were the husband of my dreams," or "I love you like no other," or "You were all I ever wanted." Heck, I'd have taken "Could you please pass me the cup of water with the bent straw?"

The tone of her last sentence to me was not something that would allow me to consider multiple hidden meanings. I'd heard that tone before. I'd heard it when I wasn't where I was supposed to be on time, "You knew this was important, and you still couldn't get here on time?" I'd heard it when I dressed the kids on Sunday morning, "You put her in that for church?" "Nooo, I just had her put that on as a stop gap between waking up and actually leaving for church! In no way did I intend for her to wear that. You think I'm an idiot?"

No, the tone was distinctly Lisa when frustrated. I'd done so many things right for her during this ordeal, and she told me as much. But this last time, whatever I did to piss her off, stuck. And unfortunately, it was the last coherent thought she shared with me.

It could have been related to me putting the oxygen mask on her face over and over and over again as she tore it off time and again in intensive care. That did make her mad. But my best guess is that her anger toward me centered around the email I sent to her doctor basically asking them not to leave her in my care over the weekend without a platelet transfusion.

Did I do the right thing? Should I have sent that e-mail? Would the outcome have been different had she stayed at home? Maybe she just wanted to die in our house, in her own bed. I haven't dwelled on her last statement to me. I know she was out of her mind, doped up on all kinds of medications. And yet, I'd give about anything for it to have been something different.

These are some of the most difficult things I would deal with as I healed from my grief. And the interesting thing is that Lisa wouldn't have done anything or said anything to hurt me had she been in her right mind. That was not her talking; at least that's what I kept telling myself.

Chapter 34

February 23 – 24, 2010

Tuesday, February 23, 5 pm

Ann stayed at the hospital with Lisa on Tuesday so that I could come home to be with the girls and to get some rest. We decided to let the girls go visit Mom if they wanted to.

I talked to each of them individually and offered them options as per the children's counselor at the KidsCan program. I told each of them that I did not know if Mom was going to live, but that she was very, very sick. I told them that they could go with me to visit her that night if they wanted to. I also told them they could draw her a picture or write her a note. I described ICU and Lisa's condition. I fully believed that each would make the right decision for them. And I was correct.

Annie T. said she did not want to go to the hospital. She wanted to draw a picture for Lisa and have me deliver it. I agreed, and she began her art project, a strong talent that she continues to refine.

Bailey too chose not to go to Duke that night. It was a very good decision for her. Several years before Lisa's illness, our former nanny, Lillian, of 11 years had a massive stroke. We went to visit her in the hospital and forced Bailey go into her room. It was a very traumatic experience for her. She got very upset. It didn't do Bailey or Lillian any good. I knew Lisa was unconscious and told Bailey that she would not be able to talk. With that being said, Bailey decided to write her a note which was sweet and appropriate for her.

Lucy, on the other hand, immediately jumped at the chance to visit her mother. There was no question in her mind that she wanted to see her. For Lucy, we could not leave soon enough.

After dinner, I collected the note and artwork and Lucy and we headed down I-40 to Duke. On the way, I reemphasized what ICU was like, that Lisa was on oxygen and that she probably would not respond to what we said. I told her I did not know what Lisa could hear but that we talked to her as if she could understand all that we said. I asked Lucy if she had any questions. She said, "Yes. I have two."

"Shoot."

"Dad, if Mom dies and something happens to you, who will take care of us?"

One of my biggest fears in losing Lisa was that something would also happen to me. The thought of my girls being raised without either parent was mindboggling. Knowing it was one of my biggest fears, I could imagine it was at the top of a fourth grader's mind.

"That is a very good question, Lucy. Before I answer it, I want to ask you a question. Can you name all of the people in the world who love you?"

"You, Mom, Bailey, Annie T., Nana, Pops, Mae, Granddaddy, Aunt Sallie, Uncle Matt, Uncle Hayes, Uncle Dash, Mel, Courtney, Carlin, Hannah, Sam, Cam, Aunt Susan…"

"And that's not all Lucy. We have many friends who love you more than you will ever know."

"Uh huh. Like the Bonds and the Walkers and the Stricklands."

"Yep."

"First of all, I don't think that anything will happen to me. I'm very strong and healthy. But if Mom dies and something does happen to me, you would go live with Nana and Pops here in Raleigh until Sallie and Matt move down here from Boston. And then you would live with them. And all of your grandparents and aunts and uncles would help raise you. And our close friends would also be there to love and support you along the way. A lot of people love you, Lucy Powell."

"OK."

"Dad, if something happens to Mom, will you get remarried?" The tears began for both of us.

This is a smart kid. The two questions she asked were the two that would most affect her future. If she became parentless, who would care for her? If I brought another woman into the house, would she love Lucy? Would she take care of her like Lisa had? Wonderful, insightful questions.

"Lucy, my number one job and the most important thing to me is my girls. I love you all so much and my focus will be to take care of you — as long as you need me. I love your mother more than any other man loves his wife; I can't imagine ever loving another woman like I do her. But if something happens to Mom, one day, a long time from now, I may want to spend some time with another woman. You will grow up and will go to college and get married and have kids of your own. I might want someone to spend some time with. But Lucy, I would never get married to someone who didn't love you very, very much. And that's not something that you need to spend time worrying about right now. Mom's still alive, and I am very hopeful that she's going to get well. And if she doesn't, me spending time with someone else would be a long time in the future. OK?"

That answer seemed to satisfy her curiosity at the time. I wish I could have been more prepared for those questions. I wish my answers had been more eloquent. I felt as though I stumbled. *Did I say the right thing?*

When it comes down to it, I think the answers lie in the relationship the four of us share. There seems to be a tremendous amount of trust between my girls and me. That honesty, that ability to be open and vulnerable through the years has built a bridge that will hopefully get us through the tough times that lie ahead. I have worked hard to parent my children and yet, I have also worked hard to befriend them. I often don't know the answers to their problems, and I admit that I don't. Our willingness to share our weaknesses, theirs to me and mine to them, gives comfort. They know that what I say is the truth. Once they hear my answer, they are able to move on.

Once at Duke we met Ann in the waiting room. My mother-in-law is incredible in these difficult situations. She escorted Lucy into Lisa's room and had the nurse prepped to greet her and answer questions. At first Lucy was nervous, but Ann began to talk about the machines that were hooked up to her mother, and she so naturally touched Lisa. Her demeanor put Lucy right at ease.

We stood by the bed, smiling and talking about silly stories of the week: the homework that wasn't getting done, the cute boy in class, Dad's inability to put clothes in the right drawers after laundry. We held Annie T.'s picture up, described it in full and put it on the table. I read Bailey's note to Lisa, and Lucy smiled. I kissed Lisa's forehead and held her hand. I can't remember if Lucy kissed her. She cried when we said goodbye and as we walked to the car. I asked her if she was glad she came. She grinned and said, "Yes, Dad."

A good decision for Lucy.

I finally fell asleep around midnight. Lucy was in bed with me, breathing heavily as usual. It felt safe to have another person in the room. I took my Ambien and finally dozed off.

At 1:30 am the phone rang. I jumped. Without answering, I knew what the call meant. Ann said, "She's on an oxygen machine. You need to come now." Hayes woke to the ring.

I called my parents, my dad answered.

"This is it. Lisa is dying. Can you come now?"

"This can't be," I heard my mom shrill in the background.

"We're getting someone to come over to be with the girls. But I don't want them to wake up without a family member in the house."

"We'll be there in two hours."

Hayes called our neighbors to come over. I wanted someone they knew better in case one of the kids woke up. I called Lisa's best friend Catherine, no answer. I called another dear friend, Melanie. "She's dying. Can you come over until my parents get here?"

"I'll be right there."

It seemed like it took the neighbors 30 minutes to get to our house. "Hayes, where are they? They live two doors down. What if we don't make it to the hospital in time?"

Ann called back, "Bring something for her to wear. I don't want her to leave the hospital in their gown."

I ran to the closet. I stood there — frozen. I wanted to move fast but I couldn't. This seemed like such a significant decision. What do you put on your 39-year-old wife the night she dies? It seemed like every article of clothing had deep, deep meaning. Lisa loved clothes; there was much to choose from. I parted the sea of Ann Taylor and immediately spotted a black dress that was stunning on Lisa. It was straight and showed her shape well. A stylish short-sleeved crop jacket took something plain and made it uniquely Lisa.

I remembered the last time she wore it: to our babysitter's wedding in October, with her bad-ass white and black high heels to match. I remember unzipping that dress after a night out and all that followed. Was I making the right decision? It was black but looked sort of summery. Would her mother approve? Did I need the shoes? Why did she keep her shoes in the boxes? Where were the shoes?

"They're here. Do you want me to drive?"

"Yes. I've got a dress and shoes. She looked so good in this dress, Hayes."

As we drove down I-40 toward Durham, I was in shock. Memories of her rushed through my head. I thought of my kids, how would I tell them? How would they respond? Could there be a harder conversation in my lifetime?

Hayes and I got there before the rest of the family. I entered the room. Lisa was peaceful. The machine was loud. It was breathing for her. Her chest would inflate and then deflate like a robot. And yet, her hands were still warm. Her fingers in mine felt just right, like they did as we drove back and forth to Duke over the past six months. I kissed her cheek and forehead. Touched her hair. She was so frail. Was this really it?

David, Sallie and Matt arrived. I remember a single bellow from Matt in the hall. Ann suggested that the family give me time with Lisa alone.

I held her arm and told her that I loved her dearly. As much as I struggled to say it, I told her she could go on, that I would take care of the girls, that we'd be OK. I didn't believe my own words and wondered if she could hear me. I wanted to kiss her again and again. Which would be my last?

The family returned. We surrounded the bed, held hands and I prayed — for a life well lived, for making a difference, for comfort and peace for us all. I knew it would be a long time before we'd feel that, and I was still so damned pissed off at God. The least He could do, the very least He could do, was to bring some sense of peace to our deep, dark turmoil.

Our nurse was in the corner of the room. When I lifted my head, I could see him crying. Later he apologized. He said he seldom saw families as close and as strong as ours.

The nurse told us that she was brain dead. He said that she had no feeling and that taking her off the machine would be painless. He warned that she would have a brief period where her natural reflexes would kick in and try to help her breathe.

I said we were ready. That it was time.

A large part of me foolishly felt that Lisa would begin breathing on her own. That she would still beat this — that she was strong — that this couldn't be real. This could not possibly be my life. It was as if I was in a play, acting out a scene with deep emotion. This could not happen to me.

The machine stopped. Lisa's body began these labored deep breaths. She would gasp deeply and then pause. Over and over and over and over again. I wondered if we had made the wrong decision. I couldn't look at her. Ann stood by her head with a wash cloth wiping her brow. She said she had been there when Lisa was born and that she would be there when she left this world. She was a rock when I could not be. Ann said I could leave the room if I needed to. I desperately wanted to, but I had promised Lisa until death do us part. I sat beside her bed in a chair and held her hand.

"I think we've made a bad decision. Why is this taking so long?"

The nurse apologized and said that her youth and strength was keeping her alive longer than most. He gave her more medicine to ease the pain.

After 30 minutes off the machine, at 4 am, Lisa took her last breath. The room was silent.

Chapter 35

My childhood

I spent the majority of my life waiting for this moment. I was raised to expect that the worst possible thing would happen. It came naturally to my mother.

I'm not sure where the paranoia came from, although my grandmother did have a tough life. Her father died of the flu when she was only five years old. He left her mother, Minnie Wright, and two brothers. They immediately moved back in with Minnie's parents, Grandma and Grandpa Hendrix.

Grandma Hendrix was a large woman with one huge bosom that covered the majority of the front of her body. I only saw one picture of her; she was big and stern - her hair pulled back in a bun, wearing a cotton dress with small flowers and an apron tucked right beneath her chest. There was no smile.

Grandpa Hendrix appeared to be a strong man, a farmer, always donning overalls. The creases in his face were deep, his skin a victim of the sun and years of stress trying to feed six kids in the early 20th century.

My grandmother was a prissy girl and one of the most beautiful women who lived in Florence, SC. Although a hard worker, her pale skin and slight frame weren't much for picking and hauling the cotton Grandpa grew on his land.

After a few years, Minnie remarried another man with the same last name as her first husband, we called him Daddy Wright. She moved in with him and left her three children with her parents on the farm.

I feel certain that this abandonment had something to do with my grandmother's inability to let my mother out of her sight. My mom didn't have that many friends growing up because she spent most of her time with her parents. She was taught to fear strangers, burglars, accidents, water, diseases, driving late at night, traveling, her own shadow. My grandmother had lost her father and then essentially her mother at a very early age; she was not about to lose her only child. Every precaution would be taken to keep her safe including not letting her leave the concentric circle of their family.

Although my mom fought hard not to pass her mother's inane fears on to my brother and me, some of them seeped into the genetic pool.

When your mother locks the door the minute you step onto the porch stoop, you begin to get the feeling that there is a high probability that someone, who isn't supposed to, is trying to get in your house. There weren't many weeks in my younger years that someone wasn't headed to a doctor's office for some reason. If there were health savings accounts back then, our balance would have been zero, always. I spent more time in a doctor's office as a child than I did at school.

My mother never slept until we arrived home at night, regardless of the hour or circumstance. Salmonella was going to attack our systems because our meat was not cooked well enough or because we'd used a knife that at some point in its existence had touched a piece of raw chicken. I think they made the atom bomb out of chicken guts. According to my mom they are deadly and every chicken in the world is likely to carry this terminal bacteria. We were doomed. Something bad was going to happen to us.

Although in shock over Lisa's death, I was not surprised that this fate had fallen upon me. I knew it was coming. My grandmother had prepared me. My mom reinforced the idea. And they were right.

As Hayes drove me home from Duke at 5 am on February 24, 2010, my mind was consumed with two divergent thoughts: "I can't believe this has happened." And "I always knew this was going to happen."

Chapter 36

February 24, 2010, 7:00 AM

I was in a daze when Hayes and I returned to our house on Dellwood Drive slightly after 5 am. My parents greeted us with hugs and tears. Every face I saw began the next influx of sorrow. The rest of the family joined us within the hour. We sat in the den, making conversation that didn't matter.

At 7, I woke Lucy and carried her up to Bailey's room. I clutched Annie T. in my arms and carried her to Bailey's bed. We sat in a circle. Tears in my eyes.

"Mom died early this morning."

Each one frozen. Tears rolling down their innocent cheeks.

"We're going to be OK. I'm here. I love you all very much. We're going to make it."

There were no questions, just tears and hugs.

Chapter 37

February 24 - 25, 2010

A very sad update, February 24, 9:38 AM
To: Friends and Family
From: Hayes

Friends-
Earlier this morning, around 4 am, my dearest sister, Lisa Ham, passed away from complications stemming from her cancer. Her awesome (word. chosen. carefully. awesome) husband, Bruce, her parents, Ann and David, her sister, Sallie, and Sallie's husband, Matt, and I were all by her side, as was John, an incredible nurse in the Duke neuro-ICU, a man who had previously been part of the medical team for the late Ted Kennedy and in whose service our family will forever be indebted.
Bruce's parents, Jean and Wayne, were at the Hams' house, where Lisa's three daughters—the sweetest, toughest kids you will ever find, who all said the perfect goodbyes they needed to their mother at the right time—Bailey, Lucy Powell, and Annie T, were all asleep in their beds in Raleigh (well, truth be told, Lucy Powell was asleep in Mommy and Daddy's bed, because she admitted she was "a little scared"). Lisa's nephew Sam, Sallie and Matt's one-year old child, slept at Lisa's parents' house two miles from

the Hams. Friends and neighbors helped watch kids and houses in the middle of the night while all the right people slid into place.

After fighting as hard as she could, Lisa left her girls, her husband, and her family in the support of you all (who she knows she has properly instructed to take care of US all).

She let her family know she was ready to go, and she did not waste time. It's a fact: she coordinated, planned, timed, and executed the perfect death. How very Lisa of her.

Lisa's family is truly indebted to the countless folks who have supported us, and we continue to feel your love and caring. We are both harrowingly saddened by Lisa's passing and continually uplifted to see what amazing friends she made in her too brief time.

At this time, we have made no plans regarding services. We will update this list and through other venues as we make decisions.

Again, thank you for all the love you have shown Lisa and all of us.

Hayes (for the Hams and the Permars).

Lisa died early on a Wednesday morning. I wanted to have the funeral the upcoming weekend. Ann was concerned we couldn't get our act together that quickly. I didn't think I could wait until the following week. It just seemed too far away. I needed to begin the process of closure.

For some reason, it was very important to me to be able to see the faces of our best friends at the funeral. I imagined a church full of people but folks I didn't know that well taking up the prime seating in the sanctuary. I wanted to be able to look to my right and left and over my shoulder and see the people I knew had been with me and would be with me for the long haul. I sent an email to about 25 families, our closest friends, asking them to sit in reserved seating. My ulterior motive was to challenge them to stand by me; my fears of walking this road alone were significant. I'd worried about this, or a similar tragedy for years and wondered how I'd step up to the plate. I felt so vulnerable. With all of the people who surrounded me, I still felt so alone.

I understood all too fully that Lisa made the majority of the friends in our life. She built our support group. With her gone, I questioned whether they'd stay. She was the most appealing part of our partnership. If Cher is gone, does anyone really want to listen to Sonny?

Sunday, Thursday, February 25, 9:04 PM
To: Our Closest Friends
From: Bruce

Dearest Friends,

Wow, what a tough, tough week for our family. I am amazed by how gracefully my wife went through this ordeal and how gracefully she finished the fight. She said goodbye to my parents and wrote notes to the girls. We shared our fears, and I was able to share a letter I wrote to her about our partnership and how accomplished I thought she was as a person. I treasure that she told me that I was the only person she would want to walk through this with—that I was the one who she wanted to be with. She constantly told me that I had the harder job—I had to move on and raise the girls and without Oxycontin. That's bull. Never once did I sense any fear in Lisa—she did not want to leave us, but she certainly did not fear what was ahead. She also made it perfectly clear that she did not want to live in the condition she was in. She was in pain and unable to be the vibrant person she was.

In addition, Lisa instructed me on "House Rules" to share with the girls. These rules included:

1. *You have to take care of each other. Bailey, you need to teach Lucy Powell how to dress; Lucy Powell, you need to teach Annie T. how to dress.*

2. *You all have to gang up on Dad to do the things that I would want you to do when he doesn't want to do them (I suspect this has to do with spending money or letting them do things outside of my watchful eye).*

3. *I want you to be the sisters who love and support each other. I want you to work hard to get along. This is very important to me. I want you to be nice to each other unlike XXXX (and then she listed several sets of siblings they were not to emulate!)*

4. *I want you to take care of your dad (I sort of suggested that one).*

She then gave me permission to remarry and asked the girls to support that decision and she wanted them to know that. How do you remarry when you start with someone like Lisa? Isn't it incredibly selfless for her to require me to write that? Something at first that I refused to do until she said for me not to make her write it herself in her condition.

I have not yet shared "Lisa's Rules" with the girls but will in time.

*You all have supported us through this journey. It is very, very important to me to be surrounded by our closest friends and most ardent supporters during this time. I feel that the church might be full and therefore want to ask you to **meet me in Memorial Hall at our church at 1:30 pm on Sunday** if you are able to attend the Memorial Service. I would like for you—our dear friends—to walk in as a group to the sanctuary at about 1:55 and sit in the front of the church where I can see you and feel your presence.*

If you agree to this "reserved seating," there is one catch. You are now required to help the girls and me through the next few years, what I anticipate being our most difficult times. It may be through an e-mail, a letter, a night out or in, but we are going to need you.

I am scared—on many levels—for what the future brings. One thing Lisa said to me a few weeks ago was that she thought the best thing we had done for our children was to build a strong support system. She said that she didn't worry about their future because of that. You are that support system.

Thank you for your love and support.

Bruce

Chapter 38

March 1, 2010

February 14, 2010, was a Sunday. At the time, I don't think I consciously thought about it being our last Valentine's Day together. Neither of us mentioned it. But I later found out, she was thinking it.

The children had made small tokens for each of us. Mine seemed more elaborate than Lisa's. It was a mobile full of red and pink hearts made out of construction paper. I think Lisa got a card. My guess as to why I was treated with more thought was twofold. One, Lisa had been so sick that they were beginning to lose touch with her. The meds had made it more difficult to communicate with her, and she often didn't feel like doing anything but sleeping.

It was all she could do to take a shower, much less to assist them with any of their needs or spend much time with them. I also believe that they knew that I would be the one they would turn to for love and support for the rest of their lives, and they wanted to make sure I was taken care of. In hindsight, I believe their choice of Valentine gifts was an indicator that they knew Lisa's time left with us was close to the end.

Lisa found enough energy to come to the table that evening for dinner. She wheeled her knap sack full of pain meds to the table and sat at her usual spot beside Annie T. I was surprised she brought a red envelope with her that had my name on it.

I remembered to purchased trinkets for the kids, a job she usually handled. After we ate, we let the kids open their presents, and I gave

Lisa the card I had purchased for her, a comical one as usual. She was so exhausted that she went right to bed after dinner while I cleaned up the dishes.

I took my unopened card and set it by my bed. I decided I'd look at it later when she was alert. That moment never came.

She continued to decline in health and other things seemed to take precedence over the next week. I saw the envelope a few times but kept waiting for her to be there when I read it.

The day she died, there it laid on my bedside table. I held it in my hand. Would it simply be signed? Did she write anything? Lisa wasn't one to share a bunch of mushy stuff. I expected I'd open it and find it utterly unamazing.

On the day after her funeral, my parents packed their car to head back home. It was a Monday morning, and the kids had returned to school. I was about to face my first day alone. Although I didn't realize it, I was not emotionally prepared less than a week after her death, to face any time in the house by myself. But I encouraged them to leave. I felt that they had done enough. That it was time.

When I realized they were about to go, I asked them to wait. I told them about the card Lisa had left and asked them to stay in the house while I opened it.

It was a white card with a pink pig on the front. The pig was holding a pink jump rope made of hearts. Printed on the front of the card was:

love iS All around yOu…
…anD lots of It is fRom me!
hAppy vaLentiNe's daY.

The inside of the card was red and it opened vertically. On the top she left me this note dated 2/14/10.

Been stuck in bed so this is it—This is a recycled card—ain't gonna lie. You are doing <u>everything</u> you need to do. I can't think of another thing I would ask of you so don't fret about that.

- 181 -

I love you very much. Always have, always will. Forever. You're going to see some awful stuff I fear and I'm very sorry about that. But don't ever think you didn't show me how much you love me. You've always been good about that and have been patient when I couldn't. I do my best. You are the husband, father, soul mate and friend that I want—never been another. I love you very much.

Lisa

It's as if she had written that card *after* she died. How amazing that I chose not to read it until almost a week after her death and two weeks after it was written. As usual, Lisa did not go on and on about her feelings, it was short and to the point. But that made it all the more poignant in its meaning to me.

She told me the two things that I most needed to hear: that I couldn't have done more to help her throughout this horrible struggle and that she loved me as much as I loved her.

All that I had read on grief suggested that many who are left behind carry guilt. Guilt about not doing enough to care for the patient, guilt about not loving them enough or about ill feelings left unresolved. I'd had many feelings throughout this ordeal, but that was not one of them. Perhaps the absence of guilt had to do with the fact that we didn't have unresolved issues. We loved each other and respected each other. We enjoyed each other's company.

Perhaps my lack of guilt had to do with this card. A message from the one I loved who told me not to worry, not to feel responsibility for the outcome. A get out of jail free card from the only person who could issue such freedom.

Although I was totally unprepared for Lisa's death, my wife knew she was going to die and wasn't about to let that keep us from living. Instead of resentment toward those who were able to stay behind, she showered them with love and offered us an invitation to move forward without her.

She gave us the gift of a clear conscience, the gift of love. And for that, I am grateful.

Chapter 39

March, 2010

I don't remember a great deal about the two weeks following Lisa's death. I do remember the depths of my sadness. I felt such pain. I felt pain in my soul. I felt pain in places; places I didn't even know were in me.

I cried, I cried out. I had never been so emotionally distraught. At times I bellowed, literally releasing my emotion through loud vocal outbursts.

Journal Entry 3-4-10

One week ago today Lisa died. I'm trying to do all the right things—working to eat, seeing a counselor, getting out of the house each day. And yet, I am so sad, so stricken with grief at times that I am struggling to figure out how to get out of bed. It is not always that intense, but at times it is overwhelming. How do I go on? Where do I find the strength? Is it in me? How could this have happened? Am I the only one aching with grief like this? Are there others? How? Why?

Journal Entry 3-7-10

My grief continues in waves. At times I feel better, navigating the new life without her. At other times I am stricken with grief. Tonight I smelled her clothes in the closet and pulled out her sexiest panties. Oh, the memories of the romance and sex—I miss her touch, her kiss, her skin, the curve of her back, her neck, I miss it all—now it is just me.

Today I lay in bed from 7–9:15 am in Fayetteville with kids climbing all over me—trying to get the strength and motivation to get up.

A week and a half after Lisa died, I went to my parents' house in Fayetteville for the weekend. Being there was as painful, if not more so, than being at home. That house with the long dining room table set for the entire family with one person so obviously missing. The family recipes passed down from my Grandmother Ham, how can butter beans make one feel sad?

My brother and his wife, he in my father's recliner, her on his lap. The intimacy they share that is gone for me — perhaps forever.

We arrived in Fayetteville on Friday afternoon. I took a nap and when awoken, I could not get out of the bed. I was paralyzed, virtually unable to move. The weekend continued like that with deep, dark despair.

The thought of returning to our house on Sunday afternoon with no plans for dinner stared me in the face. It was just dinner, but for me it was like facing a monster.

As we prepared to return home, my parents followed us to McDonald's on I-95 for lunch. My mom rode with me in my car, the girls with my dad in theirs. Mom said, "You can do this Bruce, you are strong."

"I'm really not. Lisa was strong. But what choice do I have?"

As we talked, I remembered that on Lisa's deathbed I told her that although I did not want her to leave, if she had to, she could. I told her I would take care of the girls and that I would handle things here on earth.

The thought of what I had promised Lisa haunted me that entire afternoon. I clearly wasn't living up to my word. I told her I would take care of things, and yet, I could hardly get out of bed.

It was that afternoon, somewhere between Fayetteville, North Carolina, and Raleigh, North Carolina, when I turned a corner. The grief was certainly not gone, I had just begun the process of healing. However, a light bulb went off for me that day. I had to commit myself to following through on what I had promised my wife. I essentially said I would raise my girls in a home that was not full of unhappiness. Our house had always been a fun, safe place for my children. Lisa expected that to remain the same.

I decided we would remember the good things about Lisa, but also as the human that she was – imperfect in ways. We picked on each other and laughed at each other for years. That could not stop. And we had to continue to laugh at Lisa. Her embarrassment as we pooted out loud at Target. In our family we called that Crop Dusting: you poot on one aisle and then walk away rapidly for the next customer to enjoy. "That one was for Mom!" I can see her now, exasperated with our immaturity.

The pain remained, it was grueling. But my attitude changed. I would work diligently not to let grief control my every move as it had for the past two weeks. I remembered what Lisa said about her condition, "I can't live like this." I too had to decide that my attitude set the tone for the house and would regulate how fierce this battle would be. I could not live like this either.

Rather than letting sadness control me, I had to work to control it. My girls had lost their mother, they could not also lose their father. It wasn't fair to them.

My anger at God, however, did not decrease with my new-found commitment to my girls.

Journal Entry 3-10-10

Received a card today from Gary B. "May God continue to bless you: he wrote. If this is His blessing I'd hate to see His curse.

Maybe He could bless your ass for a while, Gary! I've had enough of His blessings. "May Jesus wrap his arms around you," people say. Well why didn't He wrap them around us over the past six months? It's as if He was on vacation in Sedona looking at cactus flowers. "He won't give you more than you can handle." Well He has!

I've never said goddamn so much in my life. I'm beginning to feel good, not guilty, when it comes out. He, capital H???, has them all fooled. Not me. I now know. This is bullshit. I can handle being a single parent—all these dads around me are freaking out. I think that I, better than most, can raise three daughters on my own. It's the canyon he's left in the middle of my heart that I can't get over.

My therapist says that faith is the first to go and the last to come back. Well, it's gone.

It's interesting how different people responded to me after Lisa died. There were extremes. I spent a lot of time at Panera, a local coffee shop near the kids' school. At times I'd walk in and see someone I knew, and there was absolutely no mention of Lisa or our loss. It's as if nothing had happened.

"Well, hey, Bruce Ham! How the heck are you?"

I wanted to say, "My wife died a month ago, how in the hell do you think I am? I suck. I don't believe in God anymore, and I'm concerned that my kids will grow up to be whores due to a lack of a strong female role model. I haven't had sex in seven months, and I can't sleep. I can't listen to music without sobbing, and I don't like my therapist."

But I refrained. My pat answer, as my kids pointed out, was: "We're hanging in there."

The conversation quickly waned and the initiator departed as soon as he could get his hands on his toasted bagel.

At other times, I'd be sitting at a table checking e-mail and drinking my coffee and someone from St. Timothy's, usually a mom, would sit down with me and begin talking about how much she missed Lisa.

Sometimes it was someone I hardly knew, but the bond was instant. The connection deep. The conversation natural.

I found that a couple of times when I made reference to Lisa, sometimes with humor, it went over like a lead balloon.

Journal Entry: March 19, 2010

Went to dinner with the guys tonight. Had a good time – Fox & Hound. Mentioning Lisa stifled conversation so I didn't. Women can talk about it, men often cannot. All was good until Jon walked away to his car in the parking lot – then I lost it driving home. It flooded back—I'm home and still crying. Kids at BINGO night with Mom and Dad. On the way home; yelling at the top of my voice, "God fix this! You bring her back! I demand that You bring her back to me!" There is no God. You have no power.

"I hate you" entered my head and it's so frightening. But right now I do. I fear there is no God. I plead for a sign that He is real. I plead for a sign that she is OK and that I will see her again someday.

As the first month crept by, my mental state was slow to recoup.

Journal Entry: March 21, 2010

Tonight randomly started cleaning out some of her stuff in the medicine cabinet. Going through the two bags she's taken on every trip we've ever been on in our marriage. I've got a lump in my throat but am OK. She had 65 pairs of fingernail clippers. I may open a store, nah, think I'll keep and cherish them all. I do love that woman. I can't believe this has happened.

Journal Entry: March 24, 2010

> *One month ago my closest friend and companion died. I have always thought that anniversaries of deaths were silly. Why would March 24th be any tougher than March 23rd or 25th? It is but a number. THIS NUMBER HURTS LIKE HELL. Found a friend to grab a beer with at the PR at 4:30 – Eric Caldwell. Drank 1 1/2. When I picked Annie T. up from dance at six, she immediately said, "You look happier." WOW—she could notice I drank 1 ½ beers and it took the edge off.*
>
> *I can't believe she's gone for good. It can't be true. So many issues: Maura calling from school for me to check on Lucy, friends wanting to raise money for the girls, worrying about the in-laws, my sweet, sweet children. Must sleep, I'm exhausted. Lucy Powell in bed with me tonight. At some point must sleep by myself.*

I got a strong dose of single parenting those first few months. It was like being dropped naked in the middle of the Arctic Circle. I was unprepared to say the least. I was working diligently to be organized and balance work, loving my kids, homework assistance, finances and everything else that was coming my way.

One night I spent a full two hours after the kids went to bed going through school folders, reading teacher notes, making lists of things that had to be accomplished the next day, and working on the family calendar. I actually wrote ten checks that night and four of them were to the school for various events or projects.

Lisa took care of all of these details. I didn't read notes from the teacher. I didn't write the school checks. I hadn't registered a kid for a program in years. I couldn't even log onto the school website.

One event at school was BINGO night, an annual fundraiser. We had to register in advance for dinner and for the event itself. I completed all of the BINGO paperwork and attached a check.

The next morning when I got to work, I received an e-mail from a very sweet parent who was a volunteer at the school. She wrote:

Bruce, we received your BINGO information. You actually wrote one check, and we need two. One made out to St Timothy's School for the dinner and one made out to the St Timothy's PTA for BINGO. I'll have your original check for you on Friday. Thanks!

I didn't handle that well. My response:

You are trying to kill me.

I couldn't help myself. I simply typed that line and pressed send. And then I had a major temper tantrum about having to write two checks to the same place for one event. I went nuts alone in my kitchen. Shouting at the top of my voice, "I can't believe I have to write two goddamned checks for frickin' BINGO night!!! What the hell? It's one damned school. Son – of – a - bitch! That's the stupidest thing I've ever heard of in my entire life. Idiots! They're all idiots!"

This went on for about 20 minutes when I realized it was not the nice lady from school who was the idiot, it was me. I was losing it. The old camel saying with the straw that broke his back — well, two checks for BINGO apparently snapped my spine that night, perhaps my entire lower lumbar region.

You do and say some frightening things when you are faced with intense grief. Your moods swing. At times you lose control. One of my biggest fears over the first few months after Lisa's death was that I was going to flip out at work. There were times that I would be sitting in meetings and someone would be droning on about some senseless topic, and I would begin to feel the frustration and anger building up inside me. I would consciously think to myself, "You are going to stand up and yell SCREW YOU ALL! I'm through with this place. You guys don't understand life. You're sitting here talking about stuff that has absolutely no importance and you're wasting my goddamned time! I'm done. I'm outta here."

I'd picture myself tossing my notepad up in the air and storming out of the conference room slamming the door behind me. I'd feel the weight of the work-load immediately fall from my shoulders. I'd envision the e-mail that followed my departure:

Bruce Ham is no longer with the YMCA. He has decided to pursue other career opportunities. We wish him well in his new endeavors. The typical "that dude got fired" announcement.

These were thoughts I'd never before encountered. This was language that I wasn't used to using. These issues I'd struggle with for months on end.

Chapter 40

March – April, 2010

Journal Entry: March 28, 2010

Driving home from Fayetteville today listening to music with the kids. Realized I can never dance with Lisa again—no slow dance in my arms, no shagging which we loved to do, no awkward free dances where she allowed me to be goofy because I didn't know what to do with my arms or my legs. I've danced with many women in my life and we did it the best—knew each other's moves. I wish I had danced more. I never wanted to be one of the first on the dance floor because of my insecurities. Who was watching me? Now I regret.

I wondered to myself: Can anyone go through an experience like this with absolutely no regret? I wasn't eaten up with feelings of what I should or should not have done, but I did have some anguish. Most of it had nothing to do with the past seven months. Most had to do with how I'd lived my life with Lisa for the past 16 years. Why didn't I maximize our time on the dance floor?

I could see us at weddings. She was ready and willing to dance at any time. I was waiting to get a few drinks in me. I was waiting for someone else to start. It seemed that the guys who were willing to be the first ones on the dance floor were either pretty dang goofy or conversely, ultra cool. I didn't perceive myself as either. I sat and watched, afraid that all eyes would be on me. Afraid that folks could tell I didn't really know what I was doing out there. Maybe I was scared they could see the real me, the guy who couldn't climb the rope in PE in the ninth grade and who also didn't have that much rhythm.

If I had it to do over again, when the music started, I would grab her hand and lead her to the dance floor. I'd hold her tight for every slow dance. I'd shag my butt off. And when "Play That Funky Music White Boy" came on, I'd start moving in ways that would scar my children's psyches for life.

I didn't have regrets about how I cared for Lisa during her last months. I didn't worry about whether she knew how much I loved her. There were no major disagreements between us. We just didn't always maximize our time together. We sat dances out. We left the dance floor if we didn't like the song. We started dancing too late into the night. My biggest regret: missed opportunity.

I did not become obsessed with the small things we had not taken advantage of in our time together, but my emotions were fragile. The smallest things could set me into a downward spiral.

We owned a guinea pig which I hated with every fiber of my being. He was the bane of my existence.

As much as my children wanted us to be, we were never an animal family. Neither Lisa nor I particularly liked things that weren't human. We could take them or leave them if they belonged to others. We could only leave them if there was potential for them to belong to us.

I had dogs and cats growing up. I remember two in particular. One was a brown and black beagle our family adopted when I was in sixth grade. My parents allowed me to name him, and I decided we would call him "Booger." I was always enamored with bodily functions and boogers were no exception. I thought it would be hilarious to hear my mom stand in the driveway calling "Booger" for all the neighbors to hear. Begrudgingly, my father went along with my choice. My mom thought it was clever.

We also had a cat named "Bunny". She was beautiful, all white with pink ears. My mother and I had allergies, so she required all animals to spend the majority of their time outside, Bunny included. For years, Bunny went out each morning and returned for dinner and lounging in the late afternoons. This changed one summer day in 1981.

It was early evening and hot outside. I was in the den watching TV when suddenly I heard an intense moaning coming from the backyard. It sounded like a dying moose on Animal Kingdom. I ran outside to see what was happening. When I got to the deck, I could see Bunny pinned down by our backdoor neighbor's cat, Reagan. He had her legs spread, and he was about to deflower her. I raced over to them, Bunny screeching in fear. Reagan looked at me like I was the devil. He wasn't budging. He was about to nail the prettiest pussy in the Briarwood neighborhood, and he wasn't giving up without a fight.

I tried to kick him off to no avail. I still remember his eyes. They were mean —like the Child Catcher in *Chitty Chitty Bang Bang*. I ran for the hose, I felt responsible to protect my Bunny's virginity. He could get his kicks from the tacky Tabby down the street. Bunny would stay pure if I had anything to do with it. I stood there spraying him while he tried to mount. I shot the water right at his groin. He was pissed. It didn't take long before the hose and I won.

When he finally relented, Bunny scrambled under the deck. It took three hours to get her to come out. Eight months later, Mom gave her away because she still wouldn't go outside. She peed on the carpet several times, my mom had to get a litter box. She didn't do litter boxes. Therefore, the cat had to go. It didn't matter that we'd had her for a decade. It didn't matter that her picture was framed in our den. She didn't follow the rules. She was out.

If I recall, Reagan developed a strut after that day, similar to that of the star football player on the high school team after winning the conference championship.

Lisa and I decided early on that we were going to avoid animals as long as possible with our children. I remembered that taking care of them was a lot of work and that many times my animals paid the price of an over extended family who had more interest in the television than the dog.

Lisa despised her family dog, Precious, who apparently had issues with gas. Her parents still owned Precious when Lisa and I started dating. The smells that came out of that dog could linger in the house for hours.

As our children got older, the pressure for a pet grew. Lisa's mom had heard the pleas and wanted her grandchildren (in this case that overrode the fact that they were our children and we didn't want animals) to experience pet ownership. So for Christmas, when Bailey was about 8, she gave us a fish tank. If it had been a dog, I would have been very frustrated. But I felt I could handle a fish.

The day after Christmas, we filled the tank and headed to the local fish store. We picked out a number of fish. Two were fairly big so Bailey named one and Lucy the other: Mary and Vanessa. It wasn't very long before the smaller fish we'd purchased started disappearing. Morning by morning the school shrank until only Mary and Vanessa remained. The two seemed to live in peace until one day, three months into this endeavor, we noticed that Vanessa was swimming in circles because one of her fins had been damaged. A few days later, she was floating on the top of the tank with a big fat hole in her abdomen. I think Mary liked seafood.

Six months later on a Saturday afternoon, I walked by the tank and noticed that Mary had also met her demise. Bailey had a friend, Hannah, over and all the girls came to gawk.

At the time, I could not remember which girl had originally named Mary. Bailey swore it was her fish, and Lucy swore it was hers. I carried the corpse into the bathroom in a net. As we opened the toilet, a huge family war broke out about who was going to get to flush Mary down the toilet. The tears began for both of my daughters. I did not know which one to believe. I had no idea who named that fish — it had been over a year since we bought them. So I said, "I think, since you two can't agree on who named Mary, that Hannah should get to flush the fish."

You would have thought I had told my children that they had to eat staples for dinner for a year. They went nuts! Bailey informed me in a very loud voice, "IF I CAN'T EVEN FLUSH MY OWN FISH WHEN SHE DIES, I NEVER, EVER WANT ANOTHER ANIMAL AGAIN IN MY LIFE!!"

"You're killing me! Hannah, flush!"

I think we may have had a few hermit crabs purchased while at Myrtle Beach, but our next real pet came when Bailey turned ten. It was a guinea pig.

Bailey wanted a hamster but when she and Lisa went to pick it out, the employee at the pet store told them that hamsters were much more likely to bite than guinea pigs. So Lisa followed his lead.

They came home with a cage and all the fixins'. He was the cutest guinea pig you've ever seen, white, brown and tan spotted. He was pretty big and very tame. Lisa thought he looked like a cowboy and suggested that Bailey name him John Wayne. Bailey batted around several other names but, I think to please her mother, landed on JW. She fed him, played with him and cleaned his cage without reminders or argument, for a week. Then she lost all interest in him. When I asked her why, she said, "I didn't really want a guinea pig. I wanted a hamster. Mom made me get him. So, I don't like him."

We stayed on her about taking care of him. I had to punish her until she would clean his cage. I ended up playing with him some and feeding him often simply because I felt if I didn't, he would starve.

When we went out of town, I would get a pet sitter, and I would pay her. I had to purchase the food and shavings for his cage. I often helped Bailey clean up after him and he grew BIG, the size of a small cat. He was a pain in the butt.

When Lisa died, we had owned JW for three years and two months. I remember going into the basement the week Lisa died and looking at that damn guinea pig, "I can't believe my wife is dead and YOU are alive. This is just not right. It's just not right."

About a month later, after a weekend in Fayetteville, we returned home to find JW had passed. I called all of the girls to the basement to break the news. How would they take this after seeing their mother die? Would this bring up more emotions? More questions?

"Girls, I have something to tell you."

"OK."

"JW died."

"Where is he? Can we see him?"

"He's still in his cage."

Bailey: "Can I get a fishy now?"

Lucy: "Yuck! I ain't touchin' him."

Annie T.: "Can I go take my shower?"

And me? Balling like a baby. Sobbing as I dug the large hole for the burial, snot running down my face. For them, it was nothing. For me, it was as if I had lost my wife again. Another living thing gone from our house. More quiet; more still. And my emotions on steroids.

Journal Entry March 30

> *Cleaning out is difficult. I started with the bathroom drawers. Even parting with her toothbrush was painful. Unopened make up, a half used box of tampons – I imagine those will come in handy in this house some day.*
>
> *Her night stand and desk drawers were next. Her keys – on the heart shaped key ring she had since before we were married. Directions to a friend's house. Notes from a church meeting, she was secretary of the Long Range Planning Committee. A Valentine's Day card she gave me three years ago:*
>
> *You bring out the best in me.*
>
> *Yeah, sorry to tell you this is as good as I get.*
>
> *Happy Valentine's Day*
>
> *And a special note, on a small white square piece of paper –*
> *"Stop drinking OJ. We still got it."*

Journal Entry: April 2, 2010

On a ferry boat to Nantucket with the Permars. First trip out of town without her. Was doing ok – today's a bit harder. She should be here. I miss her so. Been talking with Ann about the in-urnment service. This is so ridiculous. I sit here alone looking out at the water. Will this be my life? Could I learn to travel alone? I have a tear running down my cheek. I'm like the Native American in the littering commercial from the 70's. Is she OK? Will we meet again? I think if I was confident this would be so much easier. I'm just not right now.

Journal Entry: April 4, 2010

There are so many things we'd do together in Nantucket. Eat outside, shop for kids clothes – went into a cute exclusive kids store today that had a 50% off sale – she'd have been all over that. I did not know what to do but felt compelled to go in because I've never seen her pass up an opportunity to shop the sale racks at a kids clothing store at the beach—ever. She'd have been all over this place. Lisa saw a sale rack as an opportunity. An opportunity to dress her kids like the in crowd for 50% off! We'd been looking for madras shorts for me—found some but without her approval I wouldn't buy them. Asked Bailey about a particular bow tie. Lisa would have given the nod and "permission" to spend 50 bucks. I didn't buy it. It seems as though I'm lost without her. She'd have loved this trip. Quaint downtown shopping, a beer at four with the family. A new exploration. She should be here.

Chapter 41

April, 2010

Life is ironic. In April of 2009, we had begun to talk about how we would celebrate Lisa's 40th birthday. It would have been on April 18, 2010. Instead of celebrating that milestone, we found ourselves at her inurnment, committing her ashes. One year before, we couldn't have imagined.

Journal Entry 4-16-10

This weekend we have a lot going on. All the progress I've made could very well dissipate. This afternoon Lisa's high school friends came over to plant a tree in the yard in her memory. Very casual. At one point I sat on the walkway on the side of the house, doubled over. The road race in her memory is tomorrow. Party, basically for her fortieth birthday, tomorrow evening and the inurnment on Sunday. I think that's the one that's got me. It just feels so final. I can reason that it isn't any worse—she's not coming back regardless of where the ashes are. But there's something about this I do NOT like.

St. Timothy's School put on a road race, *The Spring Sprint*, for five years or so. The Director of Marketing felt like it would be great exposure and that the money raised by the race should be given to a charitable organization. The first year the proceeds were given to help a child at the school who needed a kidney transplant. After that, it was given to several medical research groups.

When the proceeds from the race went to help a kid at the school, Lisa loved the idea. When the funds starting going to random causes, Lisa's love was gone. As Director of Development, she spent years trying to raise money for the school. She worked diligently on the capital campaign that brought in $3,000,000 to build their new facility. She worked to raise dollars for the school annual fund. She supported the PTA as they put on their fundraising events. So asking the school community to give in the name of marketing and handing the check to someone else drove her absolutely nuts. She could think of better ways to market the school outside of raising money for medical research.

So in October 2009, when the race committee approached Lisa to ask if the proceeds from the run could go toward cancer research at Duke in her name, Lisa found herself in a bind.

This is how the one sided conversation went when Lisa got home on that fall afternoon: "That Spring Sprint has gotten me again. They know I don't like that race, it cuts into our school fundraising. Now I'm going to be the poster child for it. They aren't putting a big picture of me on their T-shirt, I'll tell you that! That money should go to retiring the debt. Duke can raise their own money."

I just giggled and kept my mouth shut.

As Lisa dealt with her illness and realized the impact that medical research could have on a family, she warmed to the idea of the school supporting a broader vision of the community. However, she asked that they not just recognize her in the process. She made a great point - that several St. Timothy's families were dealing with cancer and that they needed to take that into consideration.

In the end, after her death, we decided to run the race in memory of Lisa Ham and other families who were dealing with cancer.

The race was on Saturday, April 17, with a record number of runners in attendance. It was a great family event, and I was excited that the money was going to cancer research at Duke. I also gave a little money to the school annual fund that year just to appease Lisa.

Our dear friend, Catherine Bond, was emphatic that we plan a 40th birthday party for Lisa. In fact, Catherine was at our house on February 13, eleven days before Lisa died, asking for permission to move forward with the party plans. Lisa agreed to the party, but her gut told her she would not be there. I wish she would have been wrong.

Ten of Lisa's girlfriends planned the event to celebrate Lisa's life. One morning in March I headed into Panera for my regular cup of joe. As I neared the counter, I saw a group of people I knew. I waved but headed to the cashier to order my coffee. As I glanced back over at the table, it dawned on me that the women sitting there had nothing in common — nothing, that is, except me. There were church friends, school friends and several other random folks from my life. Clearly, they were having a conversation about something that dealt with me.

A few minutes later, Catherine came to join me at my booth. The first thing she said was, "I don't want you to speak. I want you to listen to me." I reluctantly agreed.

She then began to discuss Lisa's group of friends' desire to ensure that I followed through with the rules she wrote the weekend before she died. In particular, they felt that I might need some help/urging to spend money on the girls for frivolity. It was no secret in our circle of friends that I was thrifty. Actually, thrifty is my word. Most would say cheap. It was their desire to throw this party and ask those invited to contribute to "The Rules Fund." This fund could be used by me to buy that special pair of expensive shoes Bailey may want to wear to the prom but that I was too cheap to splurge on. It could be used to redecorate Lucy's room as Lisa did with Bailey's room the summer before she died. Lisa actually hired a decorator to consult on a 12-year-old's bedroom! The woman picked out a rug that was so expensive, Lisa paid for it out of her own savings account and would not tell me how much it cost. To this day, none of her girlfriends will tell me what Lisa paid for that rug.

"That is the sort of thing we want you to do with the money," Catherine insisted.

I was pretty adamant that we weren't asking folks to contribute to this fund and had strong arguments.

1. I had just received a nice insurance check. Although I was nowhere near rich, this money, if invested smartly, could be a significant financial cushion to allow me to educate my girls and pay for their weddings, and a couple of cool pairs of prom shoes.

2. I had a number of friends who would be invited to this celebration who had less money than I had. I just couldn't ask them to give me cash.

3. People had done so much for our family over the past year. I used to joke that my buddy Jon was going to have to build in a monthly budget line item entitled "Ham Payment." It was just too much.

4. There were others in the world who had much greater needs than we did.

5. Although I like free money, and would gladly take my lottery winnings, as the primary bread-winner in this family, I wanted to believe that I could financially care for my kids on my own.

We strongly discussed this matter. Catherine is not a pushover. She asked me to think about "The Rules Fund," that we'd talk about it later.

In retrospect, this, like the car ride to McDonald's two weeks after Lisa died, was a turning point for me. I had been cared for by my parents for 27 years. I was the kind of kid, even in college, who loved being with my mom and dad and was reliant on them when things didn't go right. Hour-long phone conversations were not uncommon for us even into my mid-20s.

I then moved to full and utter devotion and reliance on Lisa. She was my foundation. She guided me, counseled me and made many of the decisions for our family. Not only was she a strong person, but I was, to a great extent, oblivious to family issues. That was her bailiwick, not mine.

When she became sick, our family and friends stepped in to fill in the gaps that she could not. Meals were provided for nine months. The women in our lives surrounded my children, helped me clean out their clothes drawers, transported my kids from pillar to post and shopped with us. My buddies touched base through encouraging emails or phone calls, always available for a late night beer out or on my front porch when childcare wasn't available. Now it was time for me to step up to the plate and begin taking care of myself and my girls. I wasn't sure how I would do it, but I realized it was time.

I politely declined "The Rules Fund" and began planning my wife's inurnment service. No one in the family had a desire to speak at this small gathering. Ann's only input was that we meet in the historic church building and process across the parking lot to the columbarium. The rest of the program was left to me.

I encouraged the girls to each make something to put into the column barium along with the urn of ashes. Bailey and Lucy were very thoughtful in what they made.

Bailey took a small green card and printed two photographs. One was of Lisa and one was of her. She cut out their bodies. The photo of Bailey was a bit larger than the one of Lisa and was placed in the forefront of the card. The photo of Lisa was behind Bailey. The symbolism of Lisa watching from a distance was an interesting look into a teenagers thinking of where her mother might be, perhaps right over her shoulder. Bailey made two of the cards — one to be put with Lisa's ashes and one to keep by her bed.

Lucy was on an origami kick at the time thanks to a book her Nana had given to her on our recent trip to Nantucket. Because Lisa was such a snappy dresser, Lucy made a pair of origami boots. In each boot she inserted a note. One note was to Lisa and shared how sad Lucy was and how much she missed her mother. The other was a list of things she loved about her mom. The boots were bright green and reminded me of the Uggs Lisa had purchased the previous winter.

My third child took a different tact. I reminded her for weeks that she needed to think about what she wanted to put in the box. Her attitude was sort of "I'll get it done, Dad, just chill." So two days before the service, she pulled out a piece of paper and some crayons. She drew a picture of her with her mom and wrote "I miss you, Mommy." She put the picture in an envelope and addressed it, To: Mommy, Heaven Street. Ed McLeod, our pastor, said, "You don't even need a zip code for that."

I invited about 50 people to the service. These were our closest friends and family, those who had been with us before, during and after.

Ed opened the service with a welcome, a prayer and a few words. He then offered me the opportunity to speak. I wore my sunglasses to protect myself. I thanked our friends and family for their incredible support. I then read the letter that I had written to Lisa and read to her in the hospital bed on February 20.

I explained that when Lisa and I first met and fell in love, I referred to her as "my Babes." Lisa loved that name. I remember lying by her in bed in the early years. I would scratch her back gently for long periods of time. When my arm got so tired I could no longer scratch, I would write a message on her back with my finger and she'd try to guess what I'd written. The messages often included "my Babes."

My Babes,

From the time I fell in love with you in the canoe at Camp Seafarer, until this day, our partnership and relationship has been more than I ever dreamed it could have been. I believe that we have complemented each other's strengths and weaknesses like no other couple I've seen.

You—comfortable talking to a perfect stranger in a waiting room at the dance studio.

Me—looking for you to be my companion at the dance studio so I don't have to talk to people I don't know.

You—providing the much needed wings for our children, pushing them toward independence and self confidence.

Me—kissing them, hugging them and holding them in my lap as long as they will possibly stay.

You—the shopper; Target employees know you by name.

Me—the yard man, trying endlessly to grow fescue grass, to no avail.

Me—the funny man, even in inappropriate situations or when you clearly aren't in a good mood. The funny man, a wise crack, sarcastic comment, silly made-up phrase from years' past, zany dance moves or a strange garment on my head.

You—the straight man, eye roller, zinger on occasion. You have always been able to give me as much as I give you, and I think that's one of the best parts of our connection.

Both of us with tremendous love and respect for one another, our kids, our work, our church and our community.

Obviously the best thing we've done together is to raise three of the sharpest kids in the world. Not only are they beautiful and smart but they are also wise beyond their years. They are incredibly funny and a joy to be around. They seem to have your taste and refinement and my ability to burp on command. I think all three will grow up to be strong and independent, just like you and that is good.

You are an accomplished woman: got your master's degree at night from Campbell University while at the same time popping out babies and working full time. There are those who tell me you run St. Timothy's School, and I believe them. You could organize a herd of cats, as you have at church, work, and home.

*Think about the fresh ideas you brought to Bible School and Pathfinders. Think about the amount of money raised at Saint Timothy's under your leadership. You conquered Jr. League by age 28. Think about the work you did on the Long Range Plan at church; on the class of 1988's 20th reunion, the one **you** put on for Broughton High School. In many of these instances there was a team behind the project, but **you** were the engine. And you did all of this without ever missing registration for a single summer* *day camp or Y basketball program; without ever forgetting to pick a kid up from dance; without ever missing a kid's homework assignment or a command performance as the wife of the Y guy. I talk to friends of ours, other people who have lives similar to ours and I have found that there are very few who set out to conquer life as you do.*

You work full time and run the entire household (except the yard, which you've never been in). You have been integral in our church and community work. You have laid an incredible foundation for our three daughters, and you have loved me—a tall, skinny, 12-year-old with love handles, in a 44-year-old body. Thank you.

I love you dearly,

Bruce

After reading the letter, I shared a few more thoughts.

"I think Hayes unknowingly summed up how I feel about Lisa about a week and a half after she died. He said 'I don't think I'll ever get married.' I said, 'Why?' He said, 'It's not because I'm scared of losing someone, it's because I don't think I could love someone as much as you love Lisa.'

I think at times when someone dies we have the tendency to make them a saint. Lisa would have readily admitted she was no saint and actually, I wouldn't have loved her that much if she was. We tend to think that our relationship with the person was perfect — our friendship, our connection, our marriage. Our marriage was not THE perfect marriage; but it was the perfect marriage FOR US. And I believe that I loved Lisa about as much as one person could love another."

Ed then spoke eloquently about true healing in heaven, and we ended with an a cappella hymn, "Bless Be the Tie That Binds." It was the most beautiful, yet broken, song I've ever heard in my life.

After the service, the family returned to our house to visit and reflect. Bailey disappeared. In a few minutes, my mother scooted upstairs. When she came back down, she pulled me aside.

"Bailey just started her period."

"Wow."

There are things you can learn to do as a single father with daughters. There are things you just can't. I couldn't relate. I didn't know what to say. This was one of those milestones where her mother should have been present. We had revisited our loss earlier that afternoon surrounded by our friends and family. It was made more evident when we arrived home. Their mother was gone; I was all that they had.

I slowly walked upstairs, "You okay?"

"Yeah."

"You know I love you?"

"Yeah."

"Not a big deal?"

"Nah."

On the day we inurned her mother, on what would have been her 40th birthday, my oldest daughter started her period. She was becoming a woman. And in a way, I guess, I was becoming a man.

Chapter 42

Spring 2009, Spring 2010

In August, the summer before Lisa died, we went on our second annual trip to Lake Gaston to stay with four other couples at a friend's lake house. All five of us had 12-year-old daughters.

Four out of five of the girls were in the same Y Princess tribe through the YMCA. Our group was called The Barefoot Walkers. The Y Princess program is similar to Scouts, but the father has to participate with the child. All of our kids went to St. Timothy's. These girls had built a bond that seemed to be unbreakable and that same connection was growing between their parents.

When Lisa and I arrived at the lake house, the other four couples were on the porch hootin' and hollering at us. "Come on up! Grab a beer." Although excited to be there, I assumed at our age the enthusiasm would wane at about 9 pm. Surprisingly, we took a boat ride, got to talking and actually stayed up until after 1. Perhaps it was the lack of child responsibilities; perhaps it was the Michelob Ultra.

Because we stayed up a bit late on Friday night, we were beat by 8 PM on Saturday. At one point we began joking about how boring we were which led us to recount stories from our youth. One guy mentioned an escapade in their car from years gone by. Without thinking, Lisa said, "I've never done that." Everyone in the group looked at her as if she had fallen out of a tree. Truth be told, neither had I, but I didn't necessarily think I needed to shrink my manhood by announcing it with the other four more worldly guys in the room. My maturity level took a quick jaunt back to high school although I would have probably not just sat quietly when the discussion occurred in my earlier days. I would have created a story where I'd had made out multiple times in vehicles ranging from a school bus to my grandparents' Buick LaSabre.

The next day Lisa and I had to leave before any of the other couples because we had children to collect from grandparents. As we left the lake house, I glanced at her. She knew what I was thinking.

"If you can find a place."

Man! On a Sunday morning, in the daylight, in a car, and at age 43!

When she gave me the nod, we were on a two-lane country highway. The car: my new Acura TL, not very roomy but very, very cool.

I pulled off on the first side street I could find. It looked like it would do but as I drove further, we encountered multiple houses and finally a finger of the lake.

As I headed back toward the highway, I noticed a gravel road that ran 50 feet parallel to the highway. There was a tall line of trees between that road and the highway but if someone looked closely, I'm sure he could have seen us. We pulled in. The road had not been traversed in quite some time, limbs were hanging everywhere. I was a little scared that a Halifax County sheriff might pull in behind us. But not scared enough to put the car in reverse!

When I got home, I began unpacking the car. As I walked by the polished silver finish, I noticed several scratches along the driver's side — scrapes from branches on that quiet dirt path. Normally, this would have really ticked me off. I would have blamed myself for not thinking things through more clearly. But those scratches were not vandalism or carelessness on my part. Instead, they represented my marriage: two middle aged people working to reengineer a relationship for the long haul with fun, love and excitement. It was like we were twenty again.

No, I wasn't frustrated with the scrapes, not at all; in fact, I was quite proud of us. And I was in love with my wife. Lisa and I were learning to live life to the fullest. How many times do you add something to your bucket list on a Saturday night and complete it the following morning?

I'd owned ten cars in my lifetime and the Acura TL was the car of my dreams. I'd come from my first car, a Volkswagen Fastback that cost $500 and did not have a heater, to a sporty sedan with duel temperature controls and seat warmers for my cold-natured wife.

Once I actually won a car, it was a Ford Aerostar minivan.

In high school and college, I ran a summer day camp at my church. On Wednesdays we would take all of the kids to a $1 movie at the Bordeaux Theatre in Fayetteville. One summer they had a contest where you could fill out short forms with your name and address which would enter you to win a new van. I would take some of the older camp kids who were not that interested in the movie and sit them in the back of the theatre with entry forms and pencils. I'd have them complete the forms in my name — hundreds of them. I was actually a weekly winner twice during the ten week summer. That fall my mom received a call when I was off at college.

"Is Bruce Ham at home?"

"No."

"Do you know how we can contact him?"

"He's away at school."

"Well, he has won a car."

"He's not interested." Click.

My mom actually told the guy I wasn't interested! Thankfully he called back and convinced her that this was not a hoax. She called me giggling.

"Honey, I have some news for you." Giggle, giggle, giggle.

"What is it, Mom?"

"Well, you've won a new car. But at first I told the man you weren't interested." Giggle, giggle, giggle. She wasn't as excited to tell me about the car as she was to tell me she almost passed on it.

Several months later, my parents and I drove to Charlotte, North Carolina, to pick the van up. They presented the keys to me in a packed movie theater. No one cared except my mom and dad who were sitting on the back row. In fact, I think several folks threw popcorn at me. On our way back home, after stopping for lunch, I asked my mom to drive for a while. As she was backing out of the parking place at Hardees, she ran into a lamp post and put a dent in the bumper. She giggled the rest of the way home. "That's really not funny, Mom. It's a brand new car."

After ten vehicles, mostly hand me downs, I finally bought the car I wanted – the Acura TL. It was used, but it was mine.

In my family, my dad always drove the piece-of-junk car. He would purchase the good car for my mom — she did most of the family driving. I adopted that philosophy for the first 15 years of my marriage. And had it not been for strong encouragement from my wife, I would have continued that trend this time around.

Both of our cars had high mileage. One had to go. We considered several options for a new family car. Lisa was tired of driving a minivan but liked the ease of getting in and out and the ability to cram it full of kids and stuff. She really wanted a Chevy Tahoe but it seemed too small to take a family of five, with luggage, on trips, and it was difficult to crawl into the pop-up third seat. So we simply avoided the decision. At some point, we began to consider a new sportier ride for me. I struggled with driving the newer of our two cars. But we committed to purchasing her new wheels in two years when Bailey completed the eighth grade. I was getting a new car!

We bought the Acura in Fayetteville on our way to our annual YMCA Board of Visitors meeting. This time it was being held in Charleston, South Carolina. It was the third weekend in April 2009, about four months before Lisa was diagnosed. Although work for me, it was a nice getaway with my wife.

As we cruised down the highway to my meeting in my new wheels, I thought I was tough. And at that point in life, I was. The world, like my car, was going my way.

One year later, in 2010, a year after the purchase of my TL, I was headed back to the Board of Visitors meeting. This time without Lisa.

Hayes was driving Lisa's minivan and had been for months. It was getting in progressively worse condition, and with Lisa gone, I was doing a great deal of the carpooling. I really needed a larger vehicle for myself.

On my way to Asheville, the location of the meeting that year, I drove through Chapel Hill to look for my new family mobile. This time, with much less vigor than the previous year. They had what I wanted, but the price just wasn't right.

On my way back from Asheville, almost to the exact day we bought the TL a year before, I stopped at Crown Acura in Greensboro, North Carolina, to see what they had in stock: a two-year-old Aura MDX. Still a nice car, but much larger than the TL. As I test drove, I began to share my story with Jason, the salesman. He was young and seemed empathetic. He was easier to talk to than most.

After the test drive, he called a colleague to come give me a price for my trade in. The guy opened the doors and sat in the driver's seat. He turned on my TL. The engine hummed. He dug in the glove compartment and fingered through the owner's manual. He checked under the hood and released the latch for the trunk.

As he walked around the outside of the car, he glanced down and put his hand on three scratches that marked my automobile.

"Looks like a tree branch got ya," the slim guy in navy slacks casually tossed out.

"You just can't imagine" I replied.

"That's gonna cost you $1,500."

"I understand," a huge grin overtook my sad face.

It was the best $1,500 I'd ever spent. The loss of the money was well worth the memory of that dirt road on Lake Gaston. There is not any amount of money that could replace the thought of that morning for me.

I decided to buy and began completing the paperwork. I'd sign something and Jason would take it to his boss to review. I'd then head outside to cry. I'd touch the marred paint on the side of my car.

We repeated this scenario four times until I was the last customer in the showroom. As Jason unscrewed the license plate from my old car, I began to move my belongings from the TL to the MDX. I could tell he was uncomfortable with my tears – I had moved from weeping to sobbing.

And almost to the hour, one year after I purchased the car of my dreams, I traded in an incredible symbol of our relationship. It represented her love and her desire to put me first. It acknowledged her willingness to give me something that made me feel good about myself, even if it meant she had to drive an old beat up minivan for two more years. It represented her selflessness, not surprising for my Lisa.

Chapter 43

Spring 2010

The YMCA's Y Princess program has been very special to me and my daughters. My second tribe, the one with Lucy, was called The Feathered Friends. Several of the men who have participated in this father/daughter program with me have become my closest friends.

When you camp out with a group of ten dads and their daughters several times a year, you learn a great deal about each other. On one trip, we were camping at a farm in Nash County. It was November, and I don't remember being colder in my life. There was frost on the ground at 11 pm. Our fire was roaring. Several of the dads had retired for the evening. Four of us sat around the old tractor tire rim we used to contain our fire, our girls in a tent together with flashlights telling each other ghost stories that made absolutely no sense at all.

We debated politics and shared sorted stories from our past. I was always good for some tales of naked old men in the YMCA locker room. A couple of the guys had had a few too many drinks. It did, however, help keep us warm.

At one point in the evening, my buddy Jeff pointed to the sky and began to explain, in his western North Carolina drawl, about Clark's Belt. According to him, it was a shooting star that appeared every eight minutes. He explained it could only be seen on a very clear night. For the next two hours, the four of us sat with our heads looking up, never fortunate to see it.

On Monday morning, an attorney who was in the group emailed the four late nighters. "I've spent the morning on Google looking up Clark's Belt. There simply isn't such a thing. You're an ass, Jeff!"

I think each of these men shared my pain, perhaps out of fear of what they would do if their wife passed.

One day the previous fall, Lisa and I returned from the hospital to find a front porch stocked with household staples: paper towels, Goldfish, paper plates, juice boxes, cups and utensils, and on the door, a card signed, *Your buddies from the Feathered Friends Princess Tribe.*

We took the goods inside and unpacked them in their respective cabinets. I found a package with 12 bars of soap bound together in plastic. We were out, so this was especially useful. I opened the first bar.

Several months later, as Lisa's illness progressed, I noticed that many of the bars had been taken and were being used in various showers throughout the house. I wondered to myself, *Which will last longer? The soap, or Lisa?* I grabbed one of the unopened bars and took it to the closet shoving it behind my underwear. I began to get paranoid that when the soap ran out, her life would end.

She became sicker and sicker. I realized my plan wasn't working. Maybe I had it wrong. Maybe it wasn't that she'd die when we ran out of bars. Maybe it was only related to the bar that was currently in my shower. Yes! That was it. The bar was almost used up. I immediately ran to the kitchen and grabbed a Glad Ziploc sandwich bag. I carefully placed what was left of that bar in the baggie and sealed it tight. Again, I walked to the closet and placed the bag with the other bar of soap, safely under my boxer shorts.

On March 11, 2010, I found both bars when I was down to only a few pair of clean boxers. They were as I'd left them, one unused; one in pieces and in the food storage bag. I laughed at myself. *It didn't work, you moron. Lisa is gone. Silly, silly mind games.*

Did I think her life was as minute as soap? What was I thinking? I hid soap as a method to save her life. It's absurd.

Looking back on it, I think I was just desperate. I felt helpless, unable to control any part of my life. A thought popped into my head

– which will last longer? If fate had it that Lisa would, I could certainly help extend her life by protecting the soap. As far as I was concerned, this tactic had as much merit as some of the treatments she was getting at the hospital. This appeared to be the only thing I could do to help. Therefore, I preserved the soap. How interesting.

When your prayers don't seem to be working and there's nothing left to do, hide soap. It seemed perfectly logical at the time.

Chapter 44

May 2010

Journal Entry: May 6, 2010

*Mother's Day is everywhere—On TV, on the radio, at Target,
in our devotions at the Y, church flyers in the mail—I can't escape.
I'm falling apart again.*

Prior to the loss of my wife, I never understood why people struggled with holidays. We never overdid them. We'd eat dinner together and the spouse who was being honored, be it birthday or other occasion, didn't have to cook or clean up. We'd buy a card, maybe a token present. But Father's Day nor Mother's Day were significant holidays in the Ham family. And yet, this year Mother's Day gave me a solid jolt.

I received a call from Annie T.'s teacher in April. She wanted to meet to discuss Mother's Day. I know calling me was like having to fire someone. What a horrible conversation to have to have.

We met at school in Annie T.'s classroom. We sat in a circle, in small school chairs, the dry erase board behind me. The first grade lead teacher began the conversation. She gently shared with me about the annual Mother's Day Tea Party. Annie's teacher, Mrs. Robinson, told me that they led up to the event by writing and working on crafts to celebrate their mothers. They weren't sure where to go with Annie T. this year and wanted my input. They showed me their curriculum for the next few weeks. It included answering questions about your mother which would be used to write a short paper. It included a picture of your mother and a craft specifically designed for her.

I wondered if they could just stick a dagger in my kid's chest instead of requiring her to anguish through this cacophony of motherly celebration. For a moment I considered removing my kids from school until the torture was over. But what would I do next year? And the year after? I knew they had to begin pushing through, just like me. If I was the dictator of a small country, I would have just banned Mother's Day from that point forward, perhaps even replacing it with a second Father's Day.

Deep down I knew it was unfair to expect the rest of the world to stop celebrating mothers because ours had died. But good lord, what could be worse?

They asked: Do you want her to write about you? Do you want her to write about Lisa in the past tense? Should she write about a grandmother?

I was perplexed. I had no idea what to do.

Because I didn't have the answers, I was learning fairly quickly to use my resources. I'd tapped Lisa's friends for every piece of advice from braiding hair to dress length to girl drama. This time, I thought I'd go straight to the source. Some shield their kids from these types of conversations. I did not. I knew Annie T. would have an opinion. She, not her father or her teachers, needed to resolve this predicament.

That night, I curled up in bed with Annie, our nightly ritual. As I scratched her back, I began the conversation.

"I went to school this morning to meet with Mrs. Robinson because she wanted to tell me how the class was going to celebrate Mother's Day this year." I didn't know if she would get upset. I gauged my words very carefully.

"So, they will ask the kids to write about their moms as a class assignment. Since your mom is in heaven, we need to decide who you are going to write about. You could write about me or you could write about Mom, even though she is dead. You could write about Mae or Nana or even Aunt Sallie."

She interrupted, "Dad, will we be sharing these stories at the Mother's Day Tea?"

"Yeah, I think so."

"Did you say that Nana was coming to the Mother's Day Tea this year since Mommy can't?"

"Yes. I've asked her to come."

And with a sort of exasperated tone in her voice, she belted out, "Then don't you think it makes sense that I write the story about her?"

I felt pretty stupid. "Well, yes, I guess that makes perfect sense. Let's do that, T."

And the situation was resolved. After hours and days of conversations by her teachers and school administrators, and after a day of talking the situation through with my co-workers and phone calls to both sets of grandparents, in two sentences, a 7-year-old, without trepidation, made the most logical choice of all.

Lots of grown-up time and energy put toward this, simply a waste! When I suggested that she could write about me or about Lisa she looked at me like I'd fallen out of a tree.

I could nearly see her little mind at work:

Is your butt coming to the Tea? I'm fairly certain that Mom ain't gonna be there.

If Nana is the chosen one to represent, why in the world would I write about anyone else? This isn't rocket science, Dad. Does it take a seven-year-old to figure this stuff out?

It all made perfect sense to Annie T. And, it was a very good lesson for me.

Chapter 45

May 2010

Journal Entry: May 11, 2010

> *Tonight appears to be the first where I sleep alone at home. All three kids have been rotating sleeping with me. All went to bed upstairs tonight. Walking into the room it hit me that this was significant. It's just sad. The bed feels like I'm sleeping on a football field. I slip in to my side, not even wrinkling the covers past the middle. Her soft, small pillow next to mine. I kept the lights on as well as the TV. Will sound make things better? I've opened more cards—still left from the first week she died. I've taken a sleeping pill—we'll see how it works.*
>
> *Got through Mother's Day OK. I took five girls to the beach. Penny poker, crabbing, putt-putt, a day on the beach. A fun time for the most part.*
>
> *People send me pictures of her on email. I'll see a familiar expression I've forgotten and cry and cry.*
>
> *I miss her so.*

I remember when my neighbor Jim's father died when I was a kid. Mr. Martin was in the funeral home business and always drove big dark brown Cadillacs. He took us to his mortuary one day. It was an old white house in downtown Fayetteville.

I remember the front hallway, a long curved staircase meandered from the second floor. Jim asked me if I wanted to go see the caskets.

Hell, no, I don't want to see a casket. I'm petrified right now. I'm scared your dad's gonna embalm me! Let's get the heck out of here!!!

I never liked going to the Martin's house. It may have been the fact that he dealt with the dead on a daily basis. I could picture him hauling a body up that skinny staircase, the cadaver tossed over his shoulder.

Or perhaps it was that he had an amputated leg — another thing I'd not been exposed to in my few years of life. At that age, I couldn't figure out what they had done with his limb. Why had they removed it? Was it laying around the house somewhere?

Their home was dark, curtains always pulled. He sat in a recliner, the news always on.

Although I was uncomfortable in the house prior to Mr. Martin's death, I was terrified after. I enjoyed playing with their son, and Mr. and Mrs. Martin, although older, were very nice. But something about the house gave me the willies.

My fears as a child came rushing back as I pondered maneuvering my new role as the coordinator of my daughters' social calendars. I was determined that their friends would not be fearful to come to our house. I worked hard throughout the spring to invite my kids' friends over to play or for sleepovers. I had other families to dinner so that their children would become comfortable again in our house with the safety of their parents around. I had groups of kids over so that one did not have to go it alone. I had a vision of a dark, quiet, scary house; a vision that could not be. Every night I turned on lights in every room. At least one TV on for the noise.

As Mother's Day weekend approached, I began fishing around for a way to get out of town. A friend from church offered me his beach house, and I decided that might be a good place to go. Our friends, Jon and Jill, were going to Vegas for a long weekend and asked me to keep their two daughters while they were gone. Maggie was Bailey's age, tall and slender and one of the most positive spirits around. Lindsay was Lucy's best friend and a fireball. This was seemingly a selfless act for me — five girls and one dad for an entire weekend. It was actually a welcome relief.

We all loaded up on Friday after school, me and the five amigos. Topsail Beach was where our family vacationed annually each summer. We hadn't been there since Lisa died.

It was difficult driving across the drawbridge — something we'd done many times before. We threw on a Justin Bieber tune and opened the windows. The girls belted out the words like he was in the car with them. I danced too; they didn't notice my tears.

We built castles on the beach, and I taught them to play Blackjack. We stayed up late and woke up late. It was a very good distraction.

In June, birthdays hit. Lucy invited 12 friends to her sleepover; I assumed some would be out of town since it was summer. That was not the case. I also let Annie T. have a friend over that night and Bailey invited two.

I'd never planned a birthday party for one of our kids. I had paid for the parties. I had served the cake — the one that Lisa had ordered from the grocery store right after she had the invitations printed. This was my chance to step up.

After eating pizza at a local restaurant on Hillsborough Street beside NC State's campus, we walked down to the Popsicle Shop about five blocks away. I led the pack, singing YMCA camp songs along the way, complete with hand motions.

Form the orange, form form the orange
Peele the orange, peel peel the orange
Squeeze the orange, squeeze squeeze the orange
Form potato, form form potato
Peel potato, peel peel potato
Mash potato, mash mash potato
Form banana...

People eating in outdoor cafes called out, "Go, Dad!" or "You're a brave man!" I felt like a rock star. Even the bikers at Sadlack's Bar seemed to enjoy our parade.

Both sets of grandparents accompanied us to dinner but were slow on the walk to dessert. They stayed two blocks behind, so it looked like I was the sole chaperone for 18 girls. And a fun one at that.

It felt good to sing and act stupid. It felt good to be the fun dad. I was proud that I was tackling a house full of girls.

I sent out the invitations, accepted the RSVPs. I ordered the cake and bought the refreshments. I went with the girls to pick out movies and figured out how to cram the dozen and a half into our house. That's what she would have done. Now it was my turn to take up the slack.

Chapter 46

Summer, 2010

Journal Entry: June 20, 2010

It's Father's Day—piece of crap Father's Day. My beautiful, wonderful kids and parents worked very hard to celebrate today. The girls picked out a beautiful and cool bow tie for me. They also made me a man bra, "The Bro," out of cardboard and tin foil for my "man boobs." I've been doing a lot of pushups and have tried to explain the difference in muscles and flab, even pulled up pics on the web that showed men with boobs, to no avail. To them, I have man boobs.

We went to Snyder [the church I grew up in] today for the first time since Lisa died. I thought that this would be my day, much easier than Mother's Day. I'm a great father and I'd be lauded from the pulpit along with the other dads in attendance. Instead, the main part of the sermon—or one of the main parts—was on how the main responsibility of a father is to love his wife—to be an example of a strong husband for his kids. To model a strong marriage. That's nice...IF YOUR WIFE IS ALIVE!!! I do not have a wife. I am no longer married. Not only was the actual thought of the sermon tough, but I also felt like everyone in the entire church was thinking "Oooh. I wish he wouldn't say that. I feel so *sorry for Bruce." Was everyone in the room looking at me to gauge my reaction?*

Tonight in the shower I was overcome with anger at God. I fell to my knees and called him a goddamned bastard and spat at Him. I beat on the floor of my shower. I told Him repeatedly I hated Him. And it actually felt good. I felt better.

I told him He'd better help me. What am I going to do if He doesn't? Not believe and go to hell? I'm full of shit. Cussing feels good—maybe I'll get it all out.

I had been a Sunday school teacher at our church for years. Lisa and I helped start the class for young adults at the time. It stood the test of time and the "young adults" were now in their forties.

When Lisa became sick, I stopped teaching. But several months after her death, I returned, trying to get back into the swing of life.

One Sunday during this time, I began to share about how angry I'd been at God over the past year, and I recounted the day that I cussed him out in the shower. I didn't go into great detail, but I was honest about my anger. It's a pretty accepting and moderate Presbyterian Church so I thought that the class members would understand and might even gain some insight by seeing a fairly strong believer express doubts. My hope was that I'd come out the other end with a stronger faith. I just wasn't there yet.

Some folks cried as I talked. They too missed Lisa and hated to see me hurt. Many thanked me for my honesty.

Late that afternoon, however, I received a call from a woman who was in class that morning. She was a kind soul, serving on several committees at our church and, I believe, earnestly wanting to serve God. She was also very conservative.

I answered the phone, "Hello."

"Hey, Bruce, this is Mandy from First Presbyterian."

"Oh. Hello, Mandy. How are you?"

"I'm fine, and I hope you are too."

"We're hanging in there," my pat answer to that frequent question.

"Bruce, I had something I just needed to ask you."

"Alright. Shoot."

"I was just wondering if you have accepted Jesus Christ as your Lord and Savior."

I paused. "I assume this has to do with the Sunday School lesson I taught today."

"Well, yes."

I went into full defense mode. Thankfully that was my initial reaction versus the one that followed when I got off of the phone. Had she seen my anger, she might have reported back to the church that I was a heathen of the worst kind, and I might have been excommunicated — or whatever the Presbyterian equivalent of that is.

In retrospect, I'm sure this fine woman was truly concerned about my soul and wanted to make sure I was okay. She was right to check, because I wasn't.

I was pissed at God, still am at times. I felt I had always believed in an all-powerful God, and He had let me down. Clearly, in my eyes at the time, He was either not all that powerful, or He just didn't give a rat's ass about my kids or me. Why else wouldn't He step in to save Lisa?

And prayer — we had an army passionately praying for Lisa's full recovery. His lack of response made me have to fully reengineer my understanding of conversations with God. If that many people could pray for someone and it not be acted on, we must be approaching this in the wrong manner. If everyone in the world prayed for peace, would He ignore that too?

This major life event made me take a full inventory of my belief system. And yes, along the way I cussed God out. And yes, there were times when I questioned His very existence. But through it all, I hung on to my strong belief that the God I knew, the one I loved, was a God of grace and forgiveness. He was a God with large shoulders who would allow me to cuss Him out and understand how my immense pain would push me to the brink.

It would take me months and months of anger followed by healing, again followed by anger, before I discovered that He was with me the entire time. And the way I knew He was there? I knew because I was weak, and yet, I was making it – without completely falling apart. There is no way that the Bruce Ham I knew could have accomplished that on his own. Something bigger than me had given me the strength to push through and the wherewithal to begin raising my three girls with competence, love and humor. He put people in my life who threw me up on their shoulders and carried me when I couldn't do it myself.

I wish I could have been like other Christians, the ones with the mammoth faith. The ones who did not question. But I couldn't. I had lost too much. I felt betrayed. I felt duped.

It's interesting that before Lisa became ill, I could see suffering all around me and never question why my God would allow that to happen. The day it hit me directly, my tune changed. It was too close to home to obediently accept. My pain was too great to see any good that could come from the pain. I was selfish. I was human.

As I look back on my actions toward God during that time, I feel no unease. I believe that my questions, my fears, my anger awoke something in me that I'd never experienced before. I began to see hurt all around me. I gained greater empathy for those whom I encountered on a daily basis, looking more deeply at people and working more diligently to put myself in their shoes.

The more I doubted His presence, the more obvious my weaknesses were brought to life. A simple inventory of my abilities made it clear. The realization that there was no possible way I was doing this on my own was a stronger faith builder than any Bible verse or sermon I could have heard.

God spoke to me, but in a slow and quiet way. He met me where I was – alone, sad and angry. His answer was comfort, confidence in areas where I had little experience, and the prelude to peace.

Chapter 47

Fall, 2010

The first year after Lisa died, I continued to find things that she did that I was clueless about. Not only did I not know how to track my kids' homework assignments online through their school, but I knew nothing about girls' hair or clothing or even who their dentist was.

Lisa was our family's COO. She handled everything from fingernails to hooking up the printer.

After hassling my brother-in-law throughout the first six months he lived with us about issues with my computer, Hayes told me to stop being afraid of technology. He said, "Just jump in and try things until you figure out the problem. Don't be scared. You're not going to break your computer." I decided to take that same approach with the girls.

One Saturday morning, I found Annie T. in front of the bathroom mirror, getting dressed for basketball practice at the Y. She was crying, frustrated because she couldn't braid her hair.

"I can do it," I said with confidence.

"No, you can't!" she yelled. "You don't know anything about hair! You hardly have any."

"I bet I could do it. Lucy, get in here. How do you braid hair?"

"Dad — I'll just do it."

"No, I want to learn."

Lucy then proceeded to show me how to separate three strands of hair and weave them back and forth. I took the helm. The first several attempts left lumps at various points on her head. But about the fourth time, I got it right. My first braid was a small weave on the right side of her head, just enough to keep her hair out of her eyes.

I followed my success by having a quiet conversation with my wife. *How's that, baby? I did it! Just like you!*

Not long after the hair episode, I began to get reminders from other moms at school: Don't forget to pack special snack for the holiday party for Annie T. or Do you need help getting Christmas gifts for the girls' teachers?

I sat down one night in early December to do an inventory of presents I needed to purchase for those outside of the family. As I made my shopping list, I was surprised to find that combined, my three kids had 17 teachers at St. Timothy's School. I began to add up the price of celebrating their instructors, a $10 Starbucks gift card for each would equate to nearly $200. I wasn't spending that much on Uncle Hayes for Christmas, and at the time he was their second parent. I'd seen Lisa purchase nifty notepads with catchy slogans like *The more people I meet, the more I like my cat* stenciled at the top or cute Christmas ornaments. She'd buy them on sale in the off season and save them for December. But here it was mid-month and I had nothing.

"Hayes, what in the heck are we gonna do for the teachers' gifts this year? There are 17 of them!"

We pondered and brought the subject up with the girls at the dinner table.

I'm not sure who it was, but someone suggested making hot chocolate and delivering doughnuts before school. "What if Hayes played Christmas music on his guitar?" someone added. "We could carol from class to class!" The teachers would laugh, and I'd save two hundred bucks.

The day school let out for Christmas break, we arrived at school at 7:30. With us we carried Krispy Kreme doughnuts and two large carafes of hot chocolate. As we entered each classroom, we sang a specially written version of "Jingle Bells":

Dashing through the halls
In a Lands' End uniform
Each morning you greet us
With smiles so big and warm

We thank you for the things
You teach us every day
We know that grades are coming soon
We hope we get straight A's

Oh!
Thank you, ma'am
Thank you, ma'am
Thank you, Mrs. Jones
Thanks for all you do for us
We thank you, Mrs. Jones

I watched the reaction from the teachers and the students as we paraded throughout the halls of St. Timothy's School — singing and laughing (17 times!). And for the first time, I felt like they were thinking, *That's a cool family,* not, *I feel sorry for them.*

Chapter 48

Fall 2010

Some of the most difficult moments for me the first year after Lisa's death were centered around shopping for the girls. I had never independently picked out an outfit for anyone but myself. When my girls would say they needed a dress from the Lilly Pulitzer store, I assumed it was required attire for the school social. What I didn't realize was that the "Lilly" brand was optional. Yes, a dress was required, but Lilly was not!

When my daughters and I would hit the mall together, I'd look for a chair and a TV if I could find one.

One day Bailey and I were at Southpoint Mall in Durham, NC, at the Urban Outfitters store. There was a bench in the middle of the large open room where someone could sit to try on shoes. I sat, not to try on shoes but out of boredom.

Always interested in people, I began to glance around the store. What I saw were women and teens shopping in pairs or clusters. Virtually none of them were alone. None except Bailey. These groups of shoppers were laughing. Some of the moms were politely arguing with their daughters. I was being a useless slug.

My kid is alone, and I'm sitting here doing nothing, I thought to myself. *I can do this. I like to laugh and I'm beginning to learn to spar. I've seen What Not To Wear. I can shop with my 14-year-old.*

I'm sort of a clothes horse myself, although I specialize in dress shirts and bow ties. I wondered if I could take my Joseph Banks' experience and translate it to the Outfitters.

To my surprise, I found that I really enjoyed helping Bailey lug stuff around the store, and I was not short on opinions. I found myself saying things like, "You can't wear linen after Labor Day. That's a big no-no. You'd have to save that for next summer." Sometimes I'd make stuff up just to stay in the conversation: "I like the scoop neckline on that dress. The V-neck isn't flattering to your complexion." I knew that didn't make much sense but the V looked too low-cut to me and the word complexion seemed quite "shoppy."

At one point that afternoon, Bailey was in the dressing room and handed me a black skirt she'd tried on. "I need this in a medium, the large is too big."

I headed out to the sea of cotton scouring racks for her size. It was nowhere to be found. There were smalls, larges and plenty of XLs, but not one medium in the store. I even checked the size on the mannequin which made me very uncomfortable.

I glanced at the rack and noticed they had the same skirt in purple in her size. I nabbed it and headed back to the dressing room.

"Here."

"This isn't the same color."

"Purple is the new black. Just try it. It'll look great with the scoop neck shirt."

And she did. And she liked it.

It made me sad to realize that Lisa couldn't be there to go into the dressing room with my girls to help zip them up and argue with them about the appropriateness of their dress length. Instead, they had a dorky father waiting by the door, ready to give an opinion that couldn't possibly hold any level of credibility.

"Dad, what do you think?"

"I think it is defective — your butt is hanging out. It has a negative inseam. Take it off and I'll report it to the sales clerk."

I believe over time the girls warmed to my style of shopping. They discovered that if they could tolerate my opinion for two hours, they were golden. After that point, I shut down. At two hours I was done and would agree to buy anything, regardless of the price.

Girl things were hard. The shopping, hair and fingernails were so far out of my comfort zone. The only way for me to figure it out was to jump in and participate. I could have sent them with a friend or Grandma, and I did sometimes; but I didn't want to be dependent on anyone for my girls' well-being. I didn't want them to be reliant on others either. I needed them to see me as capable, that I could provide most of what their mother had provided for them. I might not have come with much raw talent in a given area. It might have been that my tactics weren't as polished, but I learned that trying and moving with self-confidence, even when I didn't feel it inside, went a long way toward their trust in me.

I had a huge fear as I began raising my girls without Lisa. I envisioned some old women looking at my kids and shaking their heads in pity: "Ahh. Look at those girls. You know, their mother died. I guess their father is doing the best he can." No. I wanted them to be pleasantly surprised! "Look at those girls! Their dad takes better care of them than most families with two parents. Those Hams are something else! I know their mother would be so proud."

Chapter 49

Fall – Winter, 2010

That first fall and winter were the worst. On Monday, January 24, 2011, we hit the eleventh month anniversary of Lisa's death. By 2:00 that day, all I wanted to do was climb in bed. For me, the sting burned deep to my core. It could last a few hours or as long as two weeks.

The anniversary, the 24th of every month, could trigger it. Who celebrates or recognizes an 11 month anniversary of anything? We don't celebrate our 11 month birthday, not even in the first year; and yet in grief, we hang on to that day. It hits us month after month after month.

The sting can hit when a holiday is heading my way. It can hit because I find one of her feminine products in the bathroom drawer. There is no rhyme or reason. And I find myself unconsciously beginning the slide. When I realize it's coming, I can typically pin point the reason: *Oh, it's the 24th; I should have prepared.* But you can't prepare. It's subconscious. Your body instinctively realizes it's time to grieve.

They say, "It's normal." It's NOT normal for me!

Never in my life had I felt this level of pain.

Bailey was sick on that Monday. I headed home mid day to make her lunch. I checked email and knocked out a few work projects. At 1 pm, I had an hour and a half meeting that I phoned in to. I lay on the couch listening to every word, trying desperately to focus. But all I wanted, all I could think about was Lisa. The sting could be paralyzing. On the outside you could see me sitting in a meeting, having a conversation with my kid, checking email. On the inside, my mind was full. My mind was consumed with my loss.

Not only was I heartsick, but I was weary, tired to the bone.

Journal Entry October 10, 2010

Life has been a struggle the past couple of weeks. Less major grief—more a feeling of being overwhelmed by all that needs to be done. I so desperately want my kids to have the same opportunities they would have had if Lisa was alive. Hayes and I cooked and served twelve middle schoolers dinner before Bailey's school dance on Thursday. Saturday we will have Annie T.'s b'day party, a "Sleep Under" for most of the kids, but she will have two of the girls spend the night. Bailey and Lucy will each have one friend sleep over too.

In addition to them, I am such a frickin' stickler about the house and yard. I work my butt off cleaning, straightening, etc. I also want to continue Lisa's traditions of decorating for Halloween, Thanksgiving, Christmas. All just to add to an already full plate.

I'm just so tired.

At first, every little step back toward normalcy was excruciating. The first time I went to the drugstore to pick up a box of Band-Aids was hard. I cried in the grocery store when I walked past her favorite yogurt. The difficulty of each little task led me to tackle only a few at the time. And then those things got easier, dairy products became a cinch.

Grief is exhausting. I likely did less physically the first year Lisa died, and yet I was never more tired, emotionally, spiritually *and* physically. As necessary tasks became easier, I was able to add in things that were less critical or that would take more emotional energy.

If it wasn't so tragic, it might have been a good sitcom. In my desire to do everything well, to do everything as she would have done, I found time and time again I was facing questions I just didn't have an answer for. One was tights. It seemed like a small thing, but for me it was significant.

It was getting cooler and one morning we were getting ready for church. Annie T. yelled out, "Dad, I need some tights. None of these fit me."

"T., there are 16 pairs in there. Certainly one, just one, will fit."

I headed up to her room and started pulling them out, one by one.

"How's this?"

"They're off white, I need white."

"What about these?"

"Dad, they have a huge run in them."

"How'd that happen?"

"I fell in the parking lot at church last time I wore them."

"Yeah, I remember. Seems like you fall a lot when you're wearing these things. Why do tights make you fall? Bai - ley, I need your help. Why are there so many runs in these dang hose?"

"Dad, you're such a guy. You can't wear tights for more than 37 minutes without getting a run in them! That's why I don't wear them."

"What about these, Annie T.?" I asked. "Oh, I can tell those are too small." I was eager to know something she didn't.

"Grab the ends, Dad, and pull," Bailey instructed.

It was like Stretch Armstrong, the toy I'd had as a kid. Except this time, the things grew, and stayed that way. By the time we got through with them, I could have worn them.

"Holy smoke! These would fit Mama Cass!"

"Who?"

"Never mind."

Needless to say, the crotch of the tights was around her ankles by the time we walked into Sunday School, but at least I got her out the door.

It was those little things, like leggings, that were about to send me to the Dorothea Dix Mental Institute. But interestingly, it was those small wins, figuring things out with help from a kid, or a grandparent or one of Lisa's friends, that was beginning to give me the confidence I needed.

Tights - conquered. One more thing I've done without her. One more hurdle behind us. Yes! Next up: singing.

Our nightly ritual for our girls' bedtime was always to read a book, sing a song and say our prayers. I don't think that I missed any days of putting the kids to bed after Lisa died. I even remember tucking them in the day she died. We all slept in my room – Bailey and me in the bed, Lucy and Annie T. on a pallet right beside us. There was something about nighttime that seemed to bring on the grief. Perhaps the darkness, or maybe it was when the mind finally had time to wander.

In January, nearly a year after Lisa died, it dawned on me that a very important part of our nighttime routine had been lost. When Lisa got sick, we stopped singing. I'd thought about it before, but just didn't have it in me. Lisa was so musical, and when she died she took much of that with her. A year after her death, I still just stared at the cross during hymns at church, unable to participate as I used to because the emotions overtook me. I remember an afternoon commute from work crying to Earth, Wind and Fire's song, "September." That is *not* an emotional tune, and yet, I boo-hooed.

But on this particular night, as I tucked Annie T. and Lucy in bed, I began to recall our favorite bedtime tune:

Frogs jump! Caterpillars hump, worms wiggle, bugs jiggle, rabbits hop, horses clop, snakes slide, seagulls glide..."

My mom taught me that one when I was a kid. I, however, added my own flare with the kids sitting on my stomach as I hopped, wiggled and jiggled them while working through the verses. My favorite was near the end, "Deer leap"— I'd say deer and then close my eyes and count to 15 or 20 in my head, not moving a muscle. Then I'd lunge my hands toward their bellies in a surprise attack and belt out the word "leap."

They'd get so nervous during those 15 seconds, I was afraid one day I was gonna get peed on. I can remember the same anxious pit in my stomach when my dad would pull a similar stunt on me as a child.

I wanted to bring the music back, but it was so hard to do. But on this cold winter's night, something hit me. It was time. I decided to pull out a golden oldie from my Bible School days: "Ah la la la la, la la le lu ia" followed by verses that we made up: "Scratch another back scratch a back next to ya, or tickle under arm under arm next to ya."

There was a bit of laughter that night, although Lucy refused to participate until we got through the "under arm" verse.

I'm not 100% sure what moved me to bring the singing back to bedtime. I think maybe it was a combination of two things. In addition to growing my capacity for parenting, my journey brought along personal growth. As I plundered through the first year, I realized that I could handle more than I ever could have imagined. I felt that there wasn't anything that could hurt me worse than losing Lisa. Once you've had brain surgery, a finger prick is nothing. Songs at bedtime, although having the potential to drag up some difficult feelings, were nothing compared to the first time I slept alone or the first time I watched the school Christmas Pageant without Lisa. It was all becoming more about my perspective. Thanks to tights and nightly singing I was gaining control of my journey, maybe for the first time in my life.

Chapter 50

February 24, 2011

A year. A full year since Lisa died.

My counselor told me it would hit me hard, but I didn't really believe her. I missed her *all* the time.

I didn't and still don't have many vivid memories of the weeks after Lisa's death. Perhaps I was just numb to the world. I vaguely remember going to Subway a day or two after she died to buy a sandwich. I thought, *They just don't understand. How can the world be so happy, so normal, when I am so not.*

But the weeks before her death were etched in my mind, like carvings on an Egyptian tomb. I could remember everything that happened the 10 days prior to February 24, 2010. Those memories are what I feared, not the memories of her last moments on this earth. As the anniversary approached, I was beginning to relive each day leading up to her death.

I remembered the Monday, a week before she died. It was the last time she would see our children. The Wednesday before she died would have been her last night in our house. Her last shower at home. I remember calling the girls at the beach that evening to tell them Lisa was going back into the hospital. She was packing, showering and shaving her legs. That phone conversation was hard.

The next day Lisa and I had a four-hour wait for her hospital room in the lobby of Duke Hospital. Remarkably, she felt pretty well. We talked, laughed – shared. Two days later, she told my parents goodbye, "You have been good to me, and you raised a good boy."

Each day took me back. Most of the thoughts were painful.

For the anniversary, Hayes and I planned a trip to the beach, just the two of us. With the girls out of town, again at their annual winter beach trip, I couldn't face just mulling around the house. We talked, I cried. He listened, and so did I. We discussed what we believed and what we didn't.

It was a tough, tough week. A time where I learned to lean into the grief.

This was also the time when I began to diligently think about what would come of Lisa's death. I began searching for something that would not only justify what we had been through, but that would make me fully alive again. I was looking for something great to occur that could help balance out my loss. Would God help me develop an outreach to those who were struggling with grief? Could I write a book that could reach folks? Certainly her death would not be in vain.

I wanted to feel balance. God had to do something big, really big. For me, a few lunches with others who had lost their spouses just couldn't justify her death. In fact, Hayes asked me, "If Bailey grows up and the loss of her mother pushes her to become a researcher, and if she finds the cure to cancer, would Lisa's death have been worth it?" Unfortunately for me, the answer to that question was not clear. If someone offered me the opportunity to get her back or cure cancer for everyone, I wasn't sure which I would choose. And the fact of the matter was, selfishly I would have likely chosen the return of my wife. If this was the case, I doubted that there was much that could happen that could grossly change my trajectory — I was going to be a sad and lonely person who lacked significant direction for the rest of my life.

Adding that realization to the heightened sadness I was feeling at that time of year increased my anxiety. Although the sun did come back out by mid-March for me, the churning desire to seek purpose in her death had escalated. On that day, my question had not been answered, and it likely never will be.

Chapter 51

Winter 2010 – Spring 2011

When I was a kid, my family would go to South Carolina for the day once a month to visit my grandparents. Both sets lived there. It was about two hours from our house in North Carolina, a straight shot down I-95. Grandmama Ham was skinny as a bean pole and was the one who could cook, and only one of my grandmothers had that talent. Every month, she would serve us a huge helping of fried chicken, cream corn and handpicked butter beans, which we poured over white rice. Without exception, my brother and I would have gas for the entire trip back home, my mother ready to crucify us by the time we hit South of the Border, a cheesy tourist trap between the Carolinas on the I-95.

"It embarrasses me to death when three of the car windows all go down at once! Everyone passing us knows exactly what just happened," my mother scolded. Although her petite frame could handle my brother and me, I always felt bad that she was so refined and feminine, and so alone with her mannerliness in our house.

The other grandmother was also a special lady and actually my favorite grandparent. Idee (as a toddler my brother couldn't say Ivy, her given name) was the one we really talked to about life. I remember sitting at her white speckled and chrome Formica kitchen table one Saturday afternoon. It was a tradition. I was a teenager and learned to drink coffee at that very spot.

On this particular day, we had a discussion about heaven.

"Idee, what do you think heaven is like?"

"Honey, it is gorgeous," her beautiful face and big green eyes lit up. "It's like being in a huge garden with clear bright skies every day."

"What do you do there?"

"Oh, you just sit around and listen to beautiful music. The angels play their harps all day."

"What do you wear in heaven?"

"There are no clothes in heaven, baby. We leave all that stuff here."

To this day, I have a horrible vision imprinted in my head of me sitting around naked on a cloud with my also naked grandparents listening to harp music in heaven. I'm not a modest person, but if they're around, I need clothes! That is NOT my idea of eternal bliss. In fact, if I had to describe hell, it would come close to that picture.

I hope God has three piece-suits and lots of bow ties and maybe a little Kenny Chesney or Usher. I'd take Bieber over angelic harp music any day.

When Lisa died, I guess those were the only real thoughts I had about where we might be after death.

Part of the angst I felt when Lisa died was a lack of full faith in what happens next. I'd been brought up to believe in heaven, and I'd never had much of a reason to question its existence — nor to question the idea of eternal life. But God had clearly let me down. He hadn't listened to me. He wasn't who I thought He was, if at all.

I hoped that this was but a short separation from Lisa. Eternity is a very, very long time, I thought. Thirty or forty years apart must be like the blink of an eye in heaven. Time had to be different there. But the questions and doubts kept coming. I begged God to send me a sign that she was alright.

On Christmas Eve, 2010, I got my first.

I was plundering through presents in the bottom of my closet that afternoon. It was a good-sized closet, a walk-in I'd shared with Lisa. By chance, or maybe not, I glanced up at the top shelf in the corner of the 8' x 9' room. I'm sure I'd looked up there before. In fact, I remember wondering where we got the quilt that was folded neatly beside the bags and shoe-boxes stored two feet above my head.

There were multiple bags lining the top shelves of our closet. All were filled with Lisa's stuff; I just hadn't been compelled to open them before. But that day, one caught my eye and for some reason, I reached up.

When I opened it, I saw a stuffed Mickey Mouse dressed in a Santa suit.

I smiled remembering our family vacation the previous December between Lisa's radiation treatment and her surgery. Lucy bought a Minnie dressed as Mrs. Claus and Lisa said, "I hate to have a Minnie without a matching Mickey." I responded, "We don't need any more frickin' stuffed animals," and walked away to find my dad.

Apparently Lisa purchased Mickey but neglected to inform me. She was infamous about purchasing gifts well in advance. I'm sure her intent was to give it to Lucy the following year or maybe even that year. She was so sick, she just forgot.

I was a little blown away by my discovery that afternoon. It was quite a coincidence that I happened to look up, and I happened to grab that one bag on Christmas Eve - and that it happened to have a Christmas gift in it purchased by my wife months before she died. I just looked up at Heaven and sort of shook my head.

Are you talking to me baby? Is there a message here?

My personality requires proof. I am a glass half empty sort of guy. A Doubting Thomas. I like to feel, smell, touch, and see before I trust or believe in anything.

I can almost hear Lisa up in heaven:

"He really didn't mean that God. I know, I know, but he really is a good guy.

Just let me go down there one time and give him a sign; maybe that'll rein him in. He'll get better, I promise. You're gonna let him in, aren't you?"

I hope her pleas help, and the experience I had that Christmas Eve surely felt like Lisa's presence.

Thirteen months after Lisa died I had a very vivid dream about heaven. It was so real. It was one of those moments when you wake up with a racing heart because you feel like you were actually participating.

I have never remembered dreams, but this night was different.

I recall seeing a place filled with those who have died before me. Grandmama Ham was actually standing there with a plate of fried chicken. My big tall goofy friend Trey, who died at the age of 32 in a car accident, was standing there with his hand in the air — a high-five and a huge hug for me. I could hear him say, in his slow southern drawl, "You finally made it, dude."

I looked around the room and spotted Lisa. She was radiant, like the day I married her. She walked over. We didn't talk but knew exactly what the other was thinking... *Finally.*

We looked at each other, and in that one glance the years apart vanished. I reached for that hand that I'd missed so many times, and we walked down a path, just the two of us. It seemed as though this time we would never have to be apart again.

It's a vivid image, an image of deep, deep comfort. It gives me hope.

I'm not sure I was communicating with the dead that night, and I probably wouldn't admit it if I really thought I was. But something put images in my head that have given me some assurance that Lisa is OK.

But Thomas here wasn't satisfied. It wasn't but a few months later that I was begging God again for another sign — something more tangible to prove to me that she was with Him.

I have found that some of my most spiritual moments occur when I'm in my car alone. One Sunday night in the spring of 2011 found me dropping all three girls off at Lake Gaston at 11 pm. A group of their friends had gone up for a few days and a dance performance required a late arrival by the Hams. I had to work the next morning and didn't want to crash the "All Lady Lake Escape," so immediately after dropping off, I jumped back in my car and began the hour and a half trip back to Raleigh.

As I hit the back roads on my journey home, I turned off the iPod and began to pray. *God, What's this all about? Can you use this situation for good? What do you want me to do? Is it writing? Spending time with others suffering from loss? What do you have in store now? God, prove to me that she's OK. I need concrete proof. Show me!*

My request was evidence of my lack of faith, something I've struggled with ever since it was challenged.

As the drive progressed, I turned my music back on, and my mind drifted to other things.

About 20 minutes later, one of my favorite songs came on my iPod. It was a Kenny Chesney song, "Out Last Night." For the first ten years of our marriage, I cracked on Lisa for her affinity for country music. I was not a fan and had no intention of becoming one. But my persistent wife ignored my resistance. "You'll like this one," she'd say in a convincing tone. With Kenny, she was right.

I sang aloud, glad that I was alone. My iPod was on shuffle so the next song could have been Kanye West or the Cheetah Sisters, any one of hundreds of tunes I had loaded. Instead, it was another country tune Lisa had shared with me, "Roll With Me" by Montgomery Gentry, another of my favorites. A smile came across my face. I knew all of the words and again, I sang as loud as I could, a Nashville star in the making.

When "Back When I Knew It All," another Gentry tune and country Lisa recommendation, randomly followed, I started laughing. An inexplicable peace filled my soul right on I-95 South. Loud bursts of laughter paired with uncontrollable tears overtook me. I felt a connection with something I could not see. I continued to sing, my hand outstretched searching for hers like so many times before.

As the song came to a close, I wondered if this had all been a fluke. But I wanted to believe. I requested a sign, could this be it?

The next was not country. It was by Mariah Carey, "Touch My Body." It has sort of a mature theme but I really like the tune. Unfortunately, I was not very discreet when I played it, and one time when it came on in the car and my good wife was in the passenger seat, Annie T. started singing all of the words at the top of her voice. Boy, did I get a lecture! "You've been playing this song in the car with our 6-year-old?

What if she starts singing 'touch my body, throw me on the floor, tussle me around, play with me some more' on the St. Timothy's playground? How do you think Father James is going to respond to that? What *are* you thinking?" The words to the song sounded more inappropriate when verbalized with no accompaniment by an angry wife.

It only took two notes of Carey's tune for me to recognize the song. My laughter grew louder and the contentment filled me. There aren't any other four songs that had more meaning to Lisa and to me than these. And they all played consecutively on random shuffle?

Had God answered my request? Was I truly connecting with Lisa? Was this His proof?

To this day I don't know.

What I do know is that a peace like I'd never felt came over my body that night near Roanoke Rapids, North Carolina. If nothing else, it brought me joy for a period of time and real hope of what could be when my time here is done. Whatever happened also gave me hope that I will see her again, that she's watching over us right now. And somehow, that makes it easier to live.

Chapter 52

September 2011

A few months before the holidays in 2010, a question began to recur in the Ham house. I'd heard it before, but this time it held more gusto. Not only was Bailey putting on the gas, but the other two had joined in. Hayes didn't help the situation.

"Dad, we've got to try out for *A Christmas Carol* this year. Hayes said he'd do it. You know Mom would want us to. Please…?"

Ira David Wood's A Christmas Carol is a play held in Raleigh every December. It was a spoof on the original with Wood, a local celebrity, playing the eccentric main character, complete with a 70 person cast that sang and danced in multiple numbers written specifically for this adaptation. By 2011, the show was playing in both Durham and Raleigh to 25,000 local fans.

This 40 year tradition starred our own Uncle Hayes as Tiny Tim when he was six. In fact, all of my in-laws had been a part of the cast in years' past, my wife included. It had been such an important part of Lisa's childhood that she tried out with Bailey in 2005. The duo was cast and for two years sang and danced their hearts out from October through mid-December.

Although I had enjoyed going to see the production, I grew to despise it when 2/5 of my family spent four to five nights a week at rehearsal while I stayed home and cared for our two youngest daughters.

"This play is getting me down!" I'd selfishly complain. "I can't work-out, I'm bathing the kids every night, we never eat dinner together, I feel like I'm single!"

Lisa would work to share how important this production had been to her as a child and what a great opportunity it was for Bailey.

"It's a huge boost to our child's confidence. She's making friends. She's becoming comfortable in front of others. She needs this!"

In addition to explaining the value this experience was bringing to our oldest daughter, Lisa did everything she could to have things around the house set for me when I got home from work. Dinner would be planned and waiting on the stove and we'd cram it down our throats before their 7 pm curtain call. Lucy and Annie's pajamas would be set out. She even began bathing them when she got home from work so that I would have one less thing to do.

I tolerated their participation, but I never endorsed it. When they didn't get cast in the third year, likely due to Bailey's transition from adorable child to preadolescent, I was elated. Lisa emailed me at work to break the news. I ran out of my office and did a victory dance for the women in the cubicles typing away at the Y.

"My wife was cut from that dang play! Hooray! It's going to be a great fall!"

Because Bailey had participated before, she had made up her mind. "I'm trying out. You can join me or not."

I was torn. Although somewhat musical, singing and dancing in front of others was not my thing. I hadn't been in a chorus since high school and certainly didn't have the confidence to sing a solo for a tryout!

I started asking questions from people I knew who had been through the process before, "What happens at the tryout?"

I was told you stood up in front of a hundred plus people and sang a solo. Then you had to learn a short dance routine.

That confirmed it. There was no way I was participating in this ridiculous escapade.

"Daaad. Can we try out without you? Uncle Hayes said he'd do it with us." Now even my younger children were pushing me.

Damn Uncle Hayes! He isn't afraid of anything, and he's dag gone good at everything! Bastard.

I knew I'd have a mess on my hands if two of the girls got in, and one was left out. I had also heard how grueling the practice schedule was going to be. Memories of past falls began to haunt me. *What if they all got in? I'll be at home from 7-9:30 or 10 pm every single weeknight from October 1 — December 20. What in the heck will I do with that much time alone? And when will I get to see my girls?*

Hayes got the tryout information. "Hey, looks like they've changed a bit from years' past. You sign up for a 10-minute slot. Sounds to me like you don't have to sing in front of a crowd — just to those who are making the decisions on who gets in."

That piece of information took my anxiety level from a 10 to a 9. I guess every little bit helped.

As I pondered my options, one thing kept poking at my heart. Lisa was in *A Christmas Carol* with Bailey, and it was a highlight of my daughter's life. Performing on a huge stage in front of thousands of people each night boosted my kid's confidence in so many ways. It exposed her to a new set of friends and to a group of eclectic people who didn't all think and look like she did. It pushed her out of her comfort zone in a really good way. Our clingy kindergartener was becoming a confident young woman, and I wondered if the play had something to do with her internal growth.

If Lisa were alive, my other two kids would have had the same opportunity. How could I not step up to the plate? How could I let my insecurities and fears dictate their future? I'd tried so hard to fill the voids that Lisa had left. Why was this any different than learning to braid hair or pick out clothes or host a sleepover? I couldn't let my girls down. I couldn't let Lisa down.

As we pulled out of the driveway heading toward the theater for tryouts on that fall Sunday evening 18 months after we lost our wife, mother and sister, I couldn't help but be proud of my girls, of my brother-in-law and yes, even of myself.

"Turn the radio off," Hayes instructed. "Everybody, roll down your windows. I'm going to count to three, and I want each one of you to sing your solo."

"At the same time?"

"Yea! At the same time."

"But, Hayes, they're different songs!"

"Exactly!"

Epilogue

Journal Entry: September 21, 2010

It's 11:36 pm — I was headed to the shower. Got a glance of myself in the full-length mirror. Stopped. Grabbed my journal. Looking at myself, what do I see? Who am I now? Who am I becoming? I see greater strength than ever before, I'm physically stronger, emotionally stronger; a man who looks every bit of his 45 years here on earth and that used to not be the case. A man wearing an old pair of reading glasses found around the house, maybe my grandfather's. A hollowness deep in those big brown eyes; maturity and newfound wisdom; a lack of innocence; deeper creases surrounding the mouth. Look deeper, deeper, what do you see? Perhaps a stronger faith growing within.

The phrase that whacks me in the head as I look back on my journal is "a lack of innocence." Can a 40-plus-year-old man have an innocence about him? I used to.

Several years after Lisa died, I was having a conversation with a friend and she said, "You lived a charmed life Bruce Ham." She was right. And I'd like that life back.

I had no idea how deeply someone could hurt. I couldn't comprehend loss or grief. I didn't know what it was like to truly be scared or anxious or to have a mind that raced so hard you could not stop it.

But accompanying this loss of innocence is a loss of judging others, a deeper understanding and empathy for what people may be going through. It also brings a greater appreciation for the precious, simple moments that occur every single hour of every single day.

I didn't mind being innocent. It was kind of nice. But maybe having to face the realization that life is tough has really made me a better person in some ways. Wouldn't it be nice if we could all gain that wisdom, the confidence within to step up to the plate and be all God intended us to be? Or if we could find pure acceptance of others and a desire to know what someone might be facing before making assumptions? And wouldn't it be nice to figure that out without going through hell here on earth?

If I had to do it again, during my first 43 years I think I'd try harder to love others for who they are and try more earnestly to understand them. I think I'd work to appreciate the beautiful things that happen to me every day — like holding my wife's hand or listening to her sing a country song along with the radio. I'd try new things. I would seek happiness and fulfillment from within which I think would have driven me to be a better husband and a better father earlier in life.

I am indeed a better person because my wife died. At this point in my journey, the thing that makes me the saddest is that she isn't here to see the man I am becoming.

Circumstances change folks; they certainly changed me.

Elisabeth P. Ham

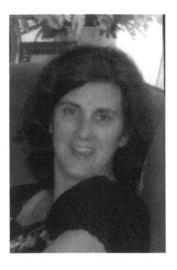

Elisabeth Hayes Permar Ham died at Duke University Hospital, Wednesday, February 24, 2010.

Lisa was born in Washington, DC, on April 18, 1970; she and her parents David and Ann Permar moved to Raleigh in 1972. She graduated from Broughton High School (1988), UNC-Chapel Hill (1992), and later received her Masters of Education Administration from Campbell University.

After college Lisa worked at the YMCA as a youth director, where her immediate supervisor, Bruce Ham, fell in love with her and asked her to marry him. At the Y she was instrumental in expanding the North Carolina Youth Legislature program, which serves teens from across the state. Lisa joined the staff of St. Timothy's School in 1994, and served as its Director of Development for 14 years, successfully coordinating the school's capital campaign for expansion and improvement of facilities.

A consummate volunteer, Lisa held several leadership positions in the Junior League of Raleigh, and served on the board of Playspace. Her commitment to First Presbyterian Church was evident through her deep level of involvement. Most recently she served on the Long-Range Planning and Building Committees, and as a Deacon. Lisa loved music and shared that love through her service as co-director of the Children's Choir. In all of her work Lisa was often the driving force to move a project forward to its successful conclusion, never seeking personal credit.

Lisa and Bruce have three daughters, Elisabeth Bailey (12), Lucy Powell (9), and Ann Truluck (7). Lisa wanted her girls to be poised and confident, to be considerate of other people, and to serve their community. She loved them as the unique individuals that they are. Lisa was a wonderful sister to Hayes Permar, Sallie Permar and her husband Matt Ferraguto, and she took great delight in her nephew Sam. She was the heartbeat of her entire family and they will miss her terribly. Some of their most poignant memories of Lisa will be during annual trips to Capon Springs & Farms, WV, and to Topsail Beach, NC. You've never experienced Disney World until you've traveled there with Lisa!

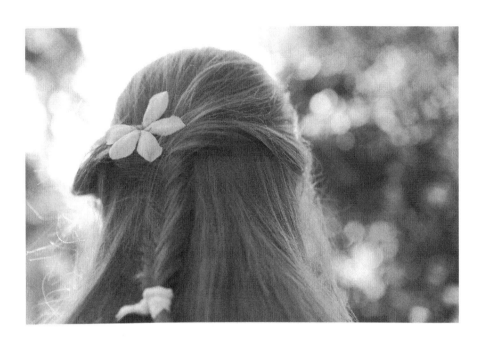

Made in the USA
Middletown, DE
09 March 2017